£41.99

Printworks Library

032199

D0421044

This item has to be renewed or returned on or before
the last date below

TWO WEEK LOAN

Library✚
Printworks Campus
Leeds City College
Book renewals & general enquiries
Tel: 0113 2846246

MILAD... ...ERIES

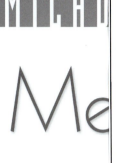

Me... ...logy

for t... ...cialist

MILADY'S AESTHETICIAN SERIES

Medical Terminology
A Handbook
for the Skin Care Specialist

PAMELA HILL, R.N.
CHRISTIAN STERLING

THOMSON
★
™
DELMAR LEARNING

Australia Canada Mexico Singapore Spain United Kingdom United States

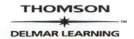

THOMSON
DELMAR LEARNING

Milady's Aesthetician Series: Medical Terminology—A Handbook for the Skin Care Specialist
Pamela Hill and Christian Sterling

President, Milady:
Dawn Gerrain

Director of Learning Solutions:
Sherry Dickinson

Acquisitions Editor:
Brad Hanson

Editorial Assistant:
Jessica Burns

Director of Production:
Wendy A. Troeger

Production Editor:
Nina Tucciarelli

Composition:
Cadmus Professional
Communications

Director of Marketing:
Wendy Mapstone

Channel Manager:
Sandra Bruce

Marketing Coordinator:
Nicole Riggi

Cover and Text Design:
Essence of 7

COPYRIGHT © 2006 THOMSON DELMAR LEARNING, a part of The Thomson Corporation. Thomson, the Star logo, and Delmar Learning are trademarks used herein under license.

Printed in Canada
1 2 3 4 5 XXX 10 09 08 07 06

For more information contact Thomson Delmar Learning, 5 Maxwell Drive, CLIFTON PARK, NY 12065-2919 at *http://www.milady.com*

ALL RIGHTS RESERVED. No part of this work covered by the copyright hereon may be reproduced or used in any form or by any means—graphic, electronic, or mechanical, including photocopying, recording, taping, Web distribution, or information storage and retrieval systems—without written permission of the publisher.

For permission to use material from this text or product, submit a request online at *http://www.thomsorights.com*

Any additional questions about permissions can be submitted by e-mail to *thomsonrights@thomson.com*

Library of Congress Cataloging-in-Publication Data

Hill, Pamela, RN.
  Medical terminology : a handbook for the skin care specialist/
Pamela Hill, Christian Sterling.
    p. ; cm.—(Milady's aesthetician series)
  Includes bibliographical references and index.
  ISBN-13: 978-1-4018-8171-9 (pbk.)
  ISBN-10: 1-4018-8171-8 (pbk.)
  1. Medicine_Terminology. 2. Dermatology—Terminology. 3. Skin—Care and hygiene—Terminology.
  [DNLM: 1. Skin—Terminology—English. 2. Cosmetics—Terminology—English. 3. Dermatologic Agents—Terminology—English. 4. Skin Care—Terminology—English.
  WR 15 H647m 2006] I. Sterling, Christian. II. Title.
  R123.H55 2006
  610.1'4–dc22
                                    2006001530

NOTICE TO THE READER

Publisher does not warrant or guarantee any of the products described herein or perform any independent analysis in connection with any of the product information contained herein. Publisher does not assume, and expressly disclaims, any obligation to obtain and include information other than that provided to it by the manufacturer.

The reader is expressly warned to consider and adopt all safety precautions that might be indicated by the activities herein and to avoid all potential hazards. By following the instructions contained herein, the reader willingly assumes all risks in connection with such instructions.

The Publisher makes no representation or warranties of any kind, including but not limited to, the warranties of fitness for particular purpose or merchantability, nor are any such representations implied with respect to the material set forth herein, and the publisher takes no responsibility with respect to such material. The publisher shall not be liable for any special, consequential, or exemplary damages resulting, in whole or part, from the readers' use of, or reliance upon, this material.

Contents

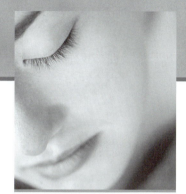

LIBRARY ✓

| CLASS NO. | 646.72 HIL |
| ACC. NO. | 032199 |

Preface

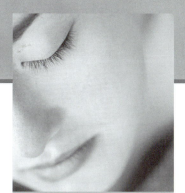

Mastering medical terminology can be a difficult feat, even for many physicians, let alone professionals in the allied medical health fields. Working with physicians and nurses can be an intimidating experience without knowing the terminology.

Because more aestheticians are found in medical offices and medical spas, it becomes increasingly important for them to have a working knowledge of the medical terminology for the context in which they are working.

Several key features separate this book from the other texts. First and foremost, *Medical Terminology* is written especially for the aestheticians of the future, emphasizing the terms that they will most often encounter "on the job."

Secondly, *Medical Terminology* contains both a refresher on the basics of language and communication, as well as an in-depth analysis of the inner workings of medical terminology. This important aspect in medical terminology is always left out. Knowing the words is one thing, but using them with ease and comfort is another story. The foundational information contained within this text—from communication to pronunciation—provides a solid platform from which to use the great amounts of valuable information that follows it.

Next, *Medical Terminology* is organized in a manner that is conducive to learning. We begin with root words, giving them ample consideration. From this beginning, we discuss prefixes and suffixes. Helpful exercises are provided, as well as an answer key to study the answers of each exercise. As with other titles in the *Milady's Aesthetician Series,* "Top 10 Tips to Take to the Clinic" highlight the key points that every aesthetician should know and remember.

Finally, Chapter 7 offers a list of pharmaceutical and cosmeceutical terms and definitions for quick reference to medications, devices, and agents common to the medical spa environment.

Good luck!

About the Authors

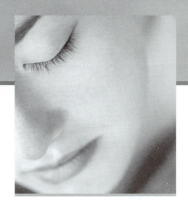

Pamela Hill, RN, CEO, received her diploma from Presbyterian/St. Luke's Hospital and Colorado Women's College. She followed through to practice as a registered nurse for more than 20 years with her initial emphasis in cardiac surgery and then in cosmetic surgery and medical skin care. In 1992, Ms. Hill founded Facial Aesthetics®, a network of medical skin care clinics in association with John A. Grossman, M.D. Since then, Ms. Hill has been an industry pioneer in the growth and development of the medical spa industry. As the president and chief executive officer of Facial Aesthetics®, Ms. Hill has been a proactive member and pioneer in the evolution of the medical spa model and the integration and union of cosmeceuticals and nonsurgical skin care. In addition to her leadership in the medical spa industry, she has also been actively engaged in the research and development of the successful Pamela Hill Skin Care product line.

Ms. Hill has devoted her passion for nonmedical skin care to the instruction of a higher level of education and skill for those aspiring to be the aestheticians of tomorrow. To further this mission, Ms. Hill founded the Pamela Hill Institute® in 2004. The goal of the Pamela Hill Institute® is to provide a uniform and comprehensive curriculum, as well as resources for aesthetic education, the advancement of cutting-edge technologies, while placing an emphasis on client care and safety for patients and students.

Christian Sterling attended the University of Colorado. In 2003 he began working for Facial Aesthetics, Inc., and has since been working in conjunction with the Pamela Hill Institute, pursuing the goals of further advancing the field of aesthetics, perpetuating uniform curriculum for aesthetics students, and assisting with the goal of quality aesthetic educational materials.

Reviewers

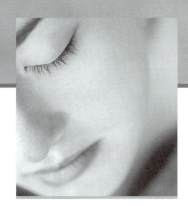

The Publisher and author would like to thank the following reviewers who contributed their insights and suggestions in the development of this book.

Alan Bunting
Loxahatchee, FL

Sallie Deitz
Bellingham, WA

Rose Palicastro
Little Ferry, NJ

Ellen Thorpe
Mesa, AZ

Acknowledgments

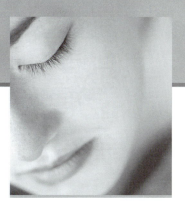

At 17, my father told me, "Be a nurse or be a teacher, you'll always get a job." I am sure he would be amazed to know where nursing has taken me. Thanks, Dad.

—Pam

To my mom for giving me life and a love of words, to George for giving me friendship, and to Pam for giving me this opportunity.

—Christian

Basics of Grammar and Speech

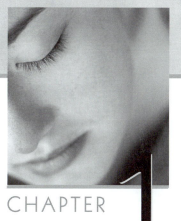

KEY TERMS

communication
encoding
idea

Indo-European family of
   languages
interpersonal
   communication

nonverbal communication
telecommunication

LEARNING OBJECTIVES

After completing this chapter, you should be able to:

1. Discuss the different types of communication.

2. Understand verbal communication.

3. Understand why English is important to medical terminology.

4. Understand the history of the English language.

5. Describe the various influences of the English language.

INTRODUCTION

From the moment we wake up to the moment we go to sleep, we exchange tens of thousands of words with people. Without the ability to do so, living in a social and orderly manner would be quite difficult. We need to communicate with one another for many reasons, of varying importance. Every part of our bodies, our senses, our mouths, and our gestures are engaged in a perpetual transmission of verbal and nonverbal codes from which we send and receive information, assign value levels, and retain (or discard) (Figure 1–1). In similar situations, different people will assign different levels of importance to the same piece of information. For example, pointing is a common form of communication in our culture; in other cultures, it is considered offensive.

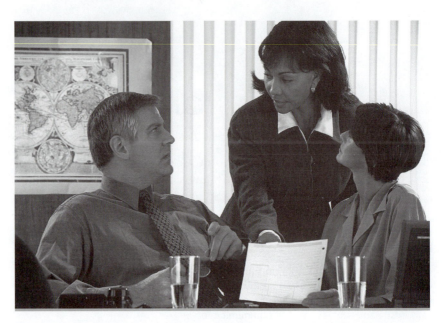

Figure 1–1 Clear communication is one of the steps to success. (Photograph courtesy of Getty Images.)

In aesthetics, the degree to which we can or cannot communicate can have far-reaching implications. These implications extend to the client's well being, your livelihood (not to mention the livelihood of your co-workers), and the overall success of the business. Failing to read signals, hear important details, and act in accordance will certainly have a bearing on the outcome of any procedure. Furthermore, in the field of aesthetics, a triangular relationship exists among the client, yourself, and the clinic. Your role will be paramount in this relationship because you will often be the go-between for the clinic and the client. You will need to act as an advocate and a representative when interacting on behalf of another. In as much, exploring the different avenues of communication will make you better prepared for clinical practice, as well as most other life situations.

However, in the clinical environment, a special type of vernacular exists, which medical professionals use to communicate, and that is medical terminology.

Why a special vernacular, you might ask? Well, simply stated, it provides a universal language of health so that health-related professionals can communicate with one another, regardless of boundaries. To get to the nitty-gritty core of medical terminology, we should first review the basics of the language, which is the universal language of medicine.

COMMUNICATION

Communication is the use of symbols to relay information. Some involve expression, some use gesturing, and some use a combination of all of these components. Contrary to what some people may believe, communication does not necessarily involve receiving. If you ask for directions from a person on the road, you have communicated with that person. Now, suppose you are in another country, and you do not speak the same language as that person on the road. Did you not communicate your need for directions, even though he or she did not understand? Consider advertising. If a commercial comes on the radio, you either listen or tune it out. The advertiser has still communicated the product or event. The mere act of sending the information is communicating.

Types of Communication

There are three primary types of communication: (1) animal communication, (2) telecommunication, and (3) interpersonal communication.

Animal Communication

Humans are not the only ones who communicate. Almost all animals use sounds (to varying degrees) to communicate with one another. Although much less understood, animals also use nonverbal communication cues as well (Figure 1–2). Cross-species communication is rare but not impossible. For example, humans and their pets are capable of communicating basic needs and emotions (Figure 1–3). Similarly, animals will rely on other animals to garner information. An example of this form of communication would be land-dwelling animals reacting to the behavior of birds in the sky or in trees to indicate the presence of a predator.

Telecommunication

We tend to think of technology or machinery when we think of **telecommunication.** Rather, telecommunications is the sending of information over large areas of space, as is the case with mass media (e.g., television, radio, motion pictures) or even smoke signals. Any form of communication that is sent to a multiplicity of persons who are separated by a distance that would make ordinary interpersonal communication ineffective is considered telecommunication. Telecommunication can be conducted by two (using a telephone or e-mail) or many more people (using television, radio, or standard mail).

communication
The use of verbal and nonverbal cues to send information to one or more people.

telecommunication
Communication over wide expanses of space.

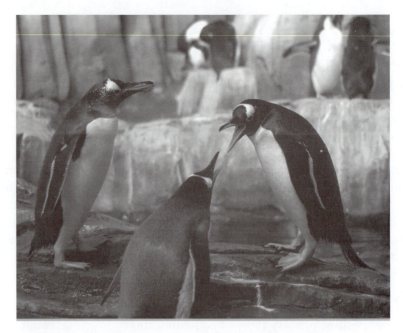

Figure 1–2 Animals communicate within the species such as this example of penguins. (Photograph courtesy of Shutterstock.)

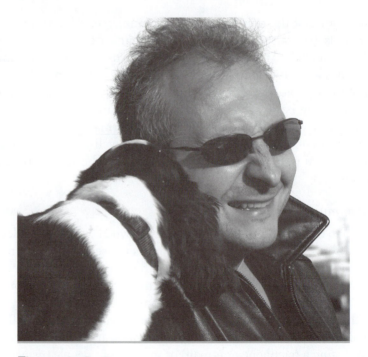

Figure 1–3 Owners and pets often have a special bond that includes communication. (Photograph courtesy of Shutterstock.)

Interpersonal Communication

Interpersonal communication, also called dyadic communication, involves communication between one person to another. This type of communication usually involves listening, dialog exchange, summarizing, paraphrasing, and gesturing. A greater instance of reception exists in this form of communication compared with other types. However, the message may not be the information the sender intended. Interpersonal communication uses both verbal and nonverbal methods.

Interpersonal communication can be conducted between as few as two people and upwards to as many as thousands. The difference between interpersonal communication and telecommunication is spatial. An instructor conducting a lecture to a thousand people in one room would be using interpersonal communication. However, if just one person is watching the lecture from a web cast, then the instructor would be telecommunicating with that one individual.

How We Communicate with One Another

Most often, we use interpersonal communication to communicate with one another. Usually, we are engaged in conversations with no more than a handful of people who are sharing a physical space. As mentioned, to accomplish this communication, we employ both verbal and nonverbal methods.

Verbal Communication

In most instances, we use words and language to send information. When a potential sender has a thought, or an **idea,** the verbal communication has its birth. For the receiver to understand the message, it needs to be encoded. **Encoding** is a cognitive process by which the sender organizes ideas into symbols. People who are adept at verbal communication will take steps to ensure that the intended recipient understands the message. To accomplish this task, words, actions, and tone are considered and chosen with the recipient in mind. The message is decoded and, ideally, received.

Verbal communication also involves the use of inflection and volume to send a message. If a person is talking in loud tones, a different meaning is conveyed than if the words are spoken in a low, monotone fashion.

Nonverbal Communication

Nonverbal communication is the process of sending a message without a verbal cue. Although nonverbal communication is usually perceived as

interpersonal communication
Communication between one individual and another.

idea
The first step to communication; ideas are translated into spoken words through decoding.

encoding
The process by which the receiver receives and extrapolates meaning from the information being communicated by another.

nonverbal communication
Communication without the use of spoken words, rather with gesturing, expression, or movement.

no, it can sometimes mean *yes*. The most common nonverbal communication is made through facial expressions. Remember that old expression, "the eyes are the window to the soul?" Your eyes are the most powerful nonverbal communicator. Your eyes can tell others what you are thinking: if you believe in yourself or if you believe the product you recommend has value. Hand gestures, body movements, touch, and personal space also play a role in nonverbal communication. Silence itself can sometimes convey information. If you are talking during a class, and your instructor stops talking and stares at you, you would easily ascertain the need for you to pay attention.

Hand gestures are an important nonverbal communication tool. If you are not warming or open to ideas, you may be bored, thus folding your arms in front of you. Some people say that folded arms also reflect a closed mind. Tapping fingers and fidgeting with your fingernails are negative nonverbal communication cues. Additionally, touching others is a nonverbal cue. The common touching technique is the squeeze of a hand or arm to offer reassurance. Similarly, hand gesturing can be used to emphasize or expand on verbal communication. If someone says something while pounding his or her fist, the intent is to emphasize the words or the emotion of the speaker. If someone is talking about the shape of a circle, drawing one in the air would be more helpful than explaining that it is a "closed plane curve everywhere equidistant from a given, fixed center."[1]

Body movements can also convey a meaning, whether implied or not or intentional or not. If someone is sitting slouched, with his or her head rested, you might assume the person is tired; or if you wanted to demonstrate respect, you may stand up when someone enters a room. Even the way you posture yourself while walking, sitting, or speaking says something in accordance with, or in opposition to, the words you use. Some people use these nonverbal cues more than they do the words themselves. How you posture yourself can tell someone how much you believe what you are saying, if you are lying, or if you know the subject about which you are talking. Self-image also plays a part in nonverbal communication. How you feel about yourself and your message will be reflected in your nonverbal cues.

Touch and personal space are important. Everyone has had the experience of being in an elevator when it is packed full of people. Being that close to people you do not know can be an uncomfortable experience. Have you ever been talking to someone and they move closer to you than is comfortable? Give people their space and respect their need to have distance from you when you talk. If someone is right in your face while they are talking, a specific meaning exists. In our culture, this posture expresses anger, or it is an intimidation mechanism; in other cultures, it is considered friendly or respectful to stand close to the person to whom you are talking. Similarly, touch can imply affection or aggression, depending of the degree of pressure applied.

HISTORY OF GRAMMAR AND SPEECH

In our culture, and in the sciences, English is the predominate language with which we use to communicate. In fact, English is on its way to becoming the world's first universal language.[2] At present, nearly a billion people speak English as a first, second, or foreign language (Figure 1–4). English is currently used as the standard for the aviation, scientific, computing, and tourism industries.

In the allied medical fields, English and medical terminology are of a common thread. When we examine the origins of the English language, we are also looking at how medical terms came to be. However, where did our language find its origins?

Indo-European Influences

English is part of the **Indo-European family of languages,** which are derived from Middle Eastern and European influences. All the subcategorized Indo-European languages are thought to have derived from a common language, for which a written record is available. The proof of

Indo-European languages
Group of languages that are derived from European and Middle Eastern influences.

Countries with English-Speaking Populations

Antigua	Grenada	St. Vincent
Australia	Guyana	South Africa
Bahamas	Ireland	Trinidad and Tobago
Barbados	Jamaica	United Kingdom (and
Belize	New Zealand	its dependencies)
Bermuda	St. Christopher	United States of
Canada	and Nevis	America (and its
Dominica	St. Lucia	dependencies)

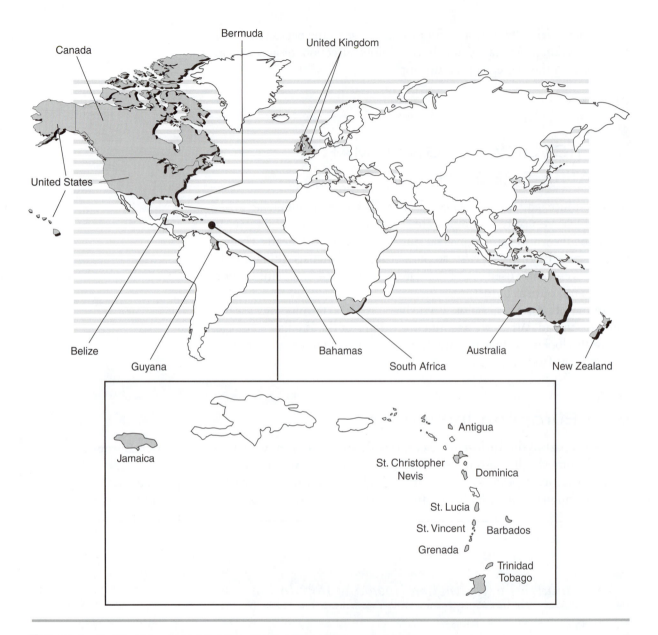

Figure 1–4 World map highlighting English-speaking countries.

this common language (called proto–Indo-European) remains in the similar words with shared meanings. For example, the words *father* (English), *Vater* (German), *pater* (Latin), and *padre* (Spanish) all have the same meaning and share a common root.[3]

> ### The Indo-European Family of Languages[4]
>
> Latin and modern Romance; Germanic
> Indo-Iranian
> Slavic
> Baltic
> Celtic
> Greek

Old English

Around the fifth century A.D., the Germanic tribes—the Jutes, Saxons, and Angles (the origin of the word *English*)—began invading the present-day British Isles. The indigenous tribes were pushed away into Scotland, Wales, and Ireland where they took their native Celtic tongue. The new inhabitants of England spoke what we refer to as Old English. The Old English was split into four dialects.

Also influencing the Old English of 900 A.D. was the northern Germanic languages, spoken by Vikings. At this time, the Vikings began invading England and intermingling their two languages.

Old England continued to expand for some time, but the Norman conquests of the British Isles soon put a halt to Old English. In fact, fewer than 10% of the known Old English words have descendants remaining today. However, they are an important 10%, including the words *be* and *water*. Most Modern English words have their origins in foreign words, mostly introduced after the Norman invasion.

Norman Invasion

The Norman invasion around 1100 A.D. is considered to be the most significant event in the evolution of the Modern English language. The native tongue of the new Norman aristocracy was French. This invasion introduced an influx of Latin-based words, spawning a period called Middle English. Chaucer spoke in Middle English.

Modern English

The Renaissance ushered in the Modern English, which we speak today. The invention of the printing press made reading materials widely available, and the English language grew exponentially. During this period, intercontinental travel became more widespread, and with that came

> The French Norman enslavement of the British had long-lasting effects on our language. Because the lower class British cooked for the Normans, we have different names for meat (veal, beef, bacon, and venison) than we do for the animals from which the meat is derived (calf, cow, swine, and deer).

many more influences that also contributed to the rapidly evolving language. One of the evolutions most noticeable today was the replacement of the *th* in some verbs, with *s* (*loveth* became *loves*; *hath* became *has*). Since then, many other languages have lent words to the English language. This list includes Latin, Greek, French, German, Arabic, Hindi, Italian, Malay, Dutch, Farsi, Sanskrit, Portuguese, Spanish, and more. The vocabulary of the English language has the largest lexicon of any language, and it is growing daily.

American English

Beginning in the 1600s, with the colonization of North America, the distinct American dialect found its place. Despite what the British may say, American English is actually closer to the English spoken by Shakespeare. When the British settled in America, they created a geographic barrier of sorts. As language evolved on the British Isles, it remained frozen in the new world. Some of the Americanisms loathed by the British are actually originally of British descent. Such words include *fall* for autumn and *trash* for rubbish. The British had forsaken these words centuries ago only to have them reintroduced in the twentieth century, thanks to Hollywood.

CONCLUSION

As the English language was evolving, so was medical vernacular. The roots, prefixes, and suffixes used in commonly spoken English are the same as are those used in medical terminology. Having a sound understanding of these components is a requirement for people who are planning on working in the allied health fields. Understanding how English, the standard medical language, evolved will help the aspiring aesthetician learn and become adept at mastering medical terminology.

▶▶▶ TOP **10** TIPS TO TAKE TO THE CLINIC

1. In aesthetics, the degree to which we can or cannot communicate can have far-reaching implications.
2. The primary means we have of using verbal communication is language.
3. In our culture, and in the sciences, English is the predominate language.
4. In the allied health fields, medical terminology is used as an industry standard.

5. In medical terminology, as in English, words have Greek, Latin, and many other languages at their root.
6. Medical terminology, as with English, is always evolving.
7. Having an understanding of the origins of the English language also helps in understanding the origin of medical terminology.
8. Body movements such as folded arms and tapping fingers can imply meaning.
9. Remember, communication may not involve receiving information.
10. Explore the intricacies of communication; doing so will make you a better clinician.

CHAPTER REVIEW QUESTIONS

1. Why is communication important to us as human beings? As aestheticians?
2. Explain the three types of communication. Which do you use most?
3. What are the characteristics of verbal communication?
4. What are the characteristics of nonverbal communication?
5. Why is English an important component of the allied medical fields?
6. What are some of the influences of the English language?

CHAPTER 1 GLOSSARY OF KEY TERMS

communication   Transmission of information by use of symbols.

encoding   Part of communication that deals with translating ideas into symbols, such as words or letters, to best enable the receiver's understanding.

idea   Beginning step of communication. Concepts and thoughts are translated into symbols and sent to the intended receiver.

Indo-European family of languages   Group of languages that are derived from European and Middle Eastern influences.

interpersonal communication   Involves communication between one person and another; also called dyadic communication.

nonverbal communication   Type of interpersonal communication whereby the sending of a message is accomplished without a verbal cue. This task is usually accomplished with hand signals, gesturing, posturing, and eye movements.

telecommunication   Communication over wide expanses of space.

CHAPTER REFERENCES

1. *Merriam-Webster's Collegiate Dictionary.* (1992). New York: Random House.
2. Katsiavriades, K., & Qureshi, T. (2002). *The English language* [Online]. Available: *http://www.krysstal.com.*
3. Katsiavriades, K., & Qureshi, T. (2002). *The English language* [Online]. Available: *http://www.krysstal.com.*
4. Katsiavriades, K., & Qureshi, T. (2002). *The English language* [Online]. Available: *http://www.krysstal.com.*

History of Medicine and Medical Terminology

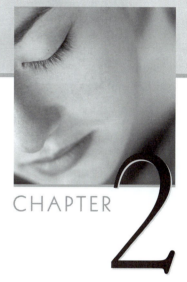

KEY TERMS

Sir Alexander Fleming
antibiotics
bloodletting
Claudius Galen
coined
computed axial
   tomography scans

deoxyribonucleic acid
dermatitis
Edward Jenner
Hippocrates
Sir Howard Walter Florey
Imhotep
Louis Pasteur

magnetic resonance
   imaging
medical terminology
prefixes
root words
suffixes
ultrasound

LEARNING OBJECTIVES

After completing this chapter, you should be able to:

1. Know a brief history of medicine.
2. Know some major contributions to the medical field.
3. Define medical terminology.
4. Understand how medical terminology works.
5. Know the history of medical terminology.

INTRODUCTION

As we have learned, as civilization has evolved, so has language and communication. Simultaneously, the field of medicine had begun and was evolving in synchronicity. In this chapter, we will examine the history of medicine and how the medical community eventually spawned its own vernacular: **medical terminology.**

medical terminology
The use of Greek and Latin roots, suffixes, and prefixes to denote diseases, conditions, and symptoms; used to create uniformity of language among medical professionals.

Imhotep
The first physician who lived in Egypt and was the pharaoh's personal physician around 2600 B.C.

HISTORY OF MEDICINE

Soon after the dawn of mankind, the most rudimentary forms of medicine began to appear. Early humans were learning the dangers of their environs and learned to avoid touching fire because it was hot; they learned to avoid poking their wounds with sticks because it would hurt; and they learned to avoid playing with saber-toothed tigers because they too would hurt. In doing so, Neanderthal man was employing preventative medicine. When humans did get hurt or become ill, they used trial and error to find remedies, when possible. Medicine would remain ignorantly dormant for thousands of years until the world's first well-structured civilizations started to examine, advance, and modernize medicine.

Medicine in Ancient Egypt

Thanks to an arid climate, papyrus documents detailing Egyptian knowledge of medicine have been well preserved. These documents revealed that most of the knowledge of medicine was rooted in myth and legend. However, Egyptians exhibited an impressive knowledge founded in human anatomy and common sense.

In Egypt, we see the advent of the physician, men whose sole job was medicine, without magic or prayer. King Zozer's personal physician, **Imhotep,** was so important during his time that he was worshipped as a god of healing following his death in 2600 B.C. (Figure 2–1).

Of most importance, the Egyptians left records indicating that they knew heart rates, pulse rates, and the significance of blood and air to the body. Some of their records actually give names to the spleen, heart, and the lungs. Undoubtedly, the Egyptians gained a vast amount of knowledge of human anatomy from their elaborate mummification processes.

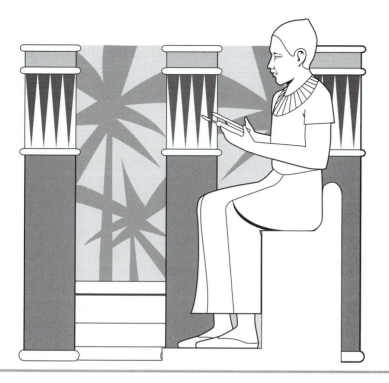

Figure 2–1 Imhotep, personal physician of King Zozer.

Medicine in Ancient Greece

A thousand years before Christ, the Greeks exhibited a detailed knowledge of the human body and its functions. Deeply spiritual, the Greeks used gods to explain almost everything. However, they were confident in their belief that illness and disease had an earthly cause and cure. Many Greek physicians were well regarded during and after the height of the Greek Empire. Most famous of these physicians is **Hippocrates.**

Hippocrates

Hippocrates (Figure 2–2) left such an indelible mark on the practice of medicine that his name is still synonymous *with* medicine. Today, physicians still take the Hippocratic Oath after completing their training. Hippocrates is also credited with highlighting the distinction between church and medicine. He argued that all work done by physicians should be done independently of the work done by a priest. Similarly, Hippocrates pioneered the belief that poor health and disease should be

Hippocrates
Greek physician who is credited with being the father of modern medicine.

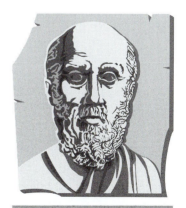

Figure 2–2 Hippocrates.

examined with reasoning and observation. He was also a strict believer that patients' experiences and feedback were critical components of diagnosis. Although evolved, the Hippocratic paradigm is still valid and practiced today.

Medicine in Ancient Rome

The Roman Civilization was well regarded for its infrastructure. Roman roads, baths, sewage systems, and aqueducts are as impressive now as they were then. Importantly, most of these architectural feats were accomplished with wellness in mind (Figure 2–3).

Medicine and wellness were first brought to Rome after assimilation of the Grecian Empire into Rome. The Greek physicians were appreciated additions to a population increasingly susceptible to illness resulting from imperialism. To combat this threat, physicians who were sprouting up in Rome argued that a healthy mind makes for a healthy body. To this avail, many Romans spent money on fitness rather than on physicians.

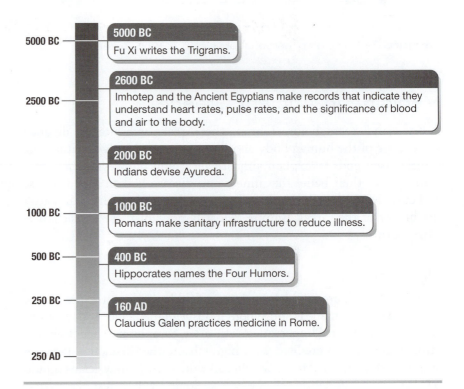

Figure 2–3 Timeline of ancient medicine.

This process worked for some, but not everyone. When scores of Romans started becoming ill with infectious diseases, the illness was traced to bad water and inadequate sewage treatment. Common information now, but we owe thanks to the Romans for this knowledge. To improve the public health, elaborate baths were erected for the lower classes and the aristocracy as well. Additionally, public toilets were built with the ever-flowing clean water supplied by the aqueducts. In essence, the Romans were the first to have a system of public health care.

Claudius Galen

Claudius Galen (Figure 2–4) is credited with reviving the teachings of Hippocrates and spreading them beyond the Greek borders, particularly into Rome, where he settled and started to practice in approximately 160 A.D. As was the case with Hippocrates, Galen placed a great deal of emphasis on clinical observation, giving each patient a thorough examination and meticulously noting symptoms.

Claudius Galen
Protégé of Hippocrates who is credited with reviving and spreading his teachings.

Galen also had an expanded knowledge of anatomy because of his dissections and subsequent documentation done on pigs and apes. He was a prodigious writer of books, believing that knowledge should be shared and expanded. His texts were still in use well into the Middle Ages during which medical research was largely abandoned until the seventeenth century.

Medical Developments in the Middle Ages

After the fall of the Greek and Roman Empires, the momentum that led to some impressive developments slowed to a virtual stop. However, by the 1300s, universities, with their sole emphasis on the instruction of medicine, began to appear. The University of Montpelier carried out the first civilly sanctioned dissection of human corpses.

The most notable characteristic of this period is the powerful direction of the Catholic Church. During the Middle Ages, the Roman Catholic Church was at the height of its glory, and it dictated the direction of medicinal study. The Church believed that illness was a punishment from God. Because any views that were in opposition to those held by the Church were considered heresy, deviations from the accepted (i.e., the Church's) position were punishable crimes. Few people deviated.

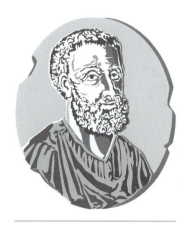

Figure 2–4 Claudius Galen.

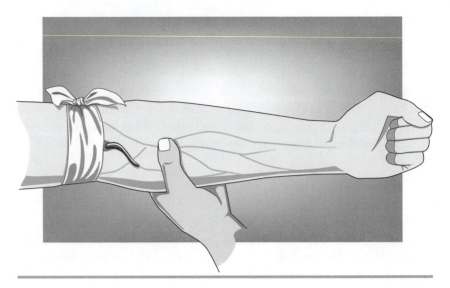

Figure 2–5 Illustration of bloodletting.

bloodletting
Early medical treatment that used released blood from the body as a means of treating disease.

Edward Jenner
British physician who discovered the vaccine for smallpox.

Treatments for illness were still primitive. **Bloodletting** (Figure 2–5) was an accepted and common practice of the time. Common thinking at that time held that most illnesses were the result of an excess of blood, and bloodletting was the obvious recourse. Veins were cut for serious illnesses, while minor injuries could be treated with leeches.

Magic and witchcraft were also more common during this period. Diagnosis and treatment were often contingent on the astrologic sign of the patient. As remedies, patients were bled or treated with herbs and potions, or both. In some instances, treatments were even more crude, drastic, and violent.

Medical Developments in the Modern Era

The modern era of medicine begins with the Renaissance in the 1600s. The Renaissance was alive with discoveries of all kinds (Figure 2–6). Knowledge, and its pursuit, was plentiful during this time. Along with such pursuits came groundbreaking discoveries that have shaped the medical field to this day. Discoveries of new diseases, cures, and techniques abounded daily.

Edward Jenner

Edward Jenner was a country physician in England. His contribution to modern medicine is a significant one. In the early 1800s, Jenner discovered a vaccination for smallpox using the less-potent cowpox. At

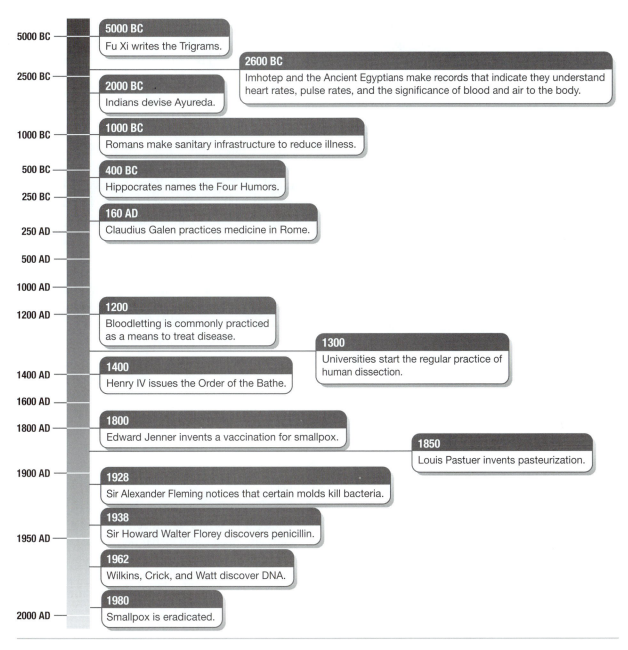

Figure 2–6 Timeline of important medical discoveries.

the time, smallpox was a pandemic that killed one in three victims, leaving the survivors disfigured. Millions of people worldwide died of smallpox to that date. After releasing the details of his discovery, Jenner was ridiculed because more urbane researchers could not believe that a physician in the countryside, without much extensive training, beat them to the punch. Jenner never patented his vaccination, saying that would make it too expensive. His was a gift that the world takes much for granted. In 1980, the World Health Organization declared the world to be free of smallpox.

Louis Pasteur

Louis Pasteur
French scientist who discovered pasteurization.

A French scientist in the middle of the nineteenth century, **Louis Pasteur** is another modern-era person who left an indelible mark on modern medicine. As most people know, Pasteur discovered that living, airborne microbes were the cause of most disease and that these organisms could be killed by heating the liquid in which they are found, preventing putrefaction. A conservative medical establishment of the time chastised him, but his discovery eventually made its way into the mainstream, bearing the name of its creator, pasteurization.

However, Pasteur's contributions did not stop there. Inspired by the works of Edward Jenner, Pasteur also discovered the vaccinations for chicken cholera, anthrax, and rabies, saving millions of lives since that time.

Sir Alexander Fleming
Scottish physician and researcher who first discovered the ability of mold to kill bacteria.

Sir Howard Walter Florey
Researcher who discovered penicillin.

Sir Alexander Fleming and Sir Howard Walter Florey

The greatest advancement to date in the treatment of disease was discovered by **Sir Alexander Fleming** in 1928. Purely by mistake, Fleming realized that a plate of staphylococcus had been killed by some mold that had grown on the plate. Ten years later, a scientist at Oxford University, **Sir Howard Walter Florey,** discovered that the substance in the mold that was capable of killing the bacteria was penicillin. In 1945, Fleming and Florey won the Nobel Prize for Medicine, and the era of **antibiotics** had begun.

antibiotics
Class of drugs that kill bacteria.

deoxyribonucleic acid
The long, double strand of genetic information, known as DNA, contained within the cells; discovered by Wilkins, Crick, and Watt.

Medical Changes Since 1945

After several hundred years of warming up, the medical field exploded in the second half of the twentieth century. Advancements were made in disease control, disease treatment, drugs, and instruments that have vastly expanded on prior medical knowledge and made medicine a much more reliable science than it was a century before.

One such advancement was the discovery of **deoxyribonucleic acid** (DNA) by Wilkins, Crick, and Watt. With the discovery of DNA, and the chromosomes contained within, science edged closer toward finding the genetic link to many diseases and illness that have plagued mankind.

With the success of penicillin, drug companies began extensively investing into research and development. Notably, hundreds more antibiotics have treated and cured thousands of diseases. Aside from antibiotics, many other drugs were developed and used to treat illnesses such as tuberculosis successfully. Today, pharmaceutical companies and medical researchers have been focusing on finding remedies to potentially fatal diseases such as Alzheimer's disease, human immunodeficiency virus (HIV), acquired immune deficiency syndrome (AIDS), and cancer.

In particular, far more surgical techniques have been discovered since 1945. More complex surgeries are being successfully completed every day. Transplants, a procedure once considered impossible, are done with regularity. Exciting and revolutionary transplant procedures are being experimented with right now. On the horizon are stem cell transplants to rebuild new tissue, facial transplants for people who are horribly disfigured by fire or accidents, and limb transplants for amputees. Another type of surgery has seen its birth during this time as well. Cosmetic or plastic surgery has gone from crude beginnings to a reliable option for people who want to improve the way they look.

Birthing and birth control have been revolutionized as well. Fertility treatments can help women who thought they could never conceive. To this avail, artificial insemination has proven most useful. Many new birth control techniques have come onto the market to aid people who do not want to conceive (some with great success, some without). Women who do become pregnant have been afforded the right to terminate unwanted pregnancies. Pregnancies can be easier for the mother with enhanced prenatal care, including amniocentesis. Birthing has also become easier with the use of epidural anesthesia. If a child is born prematurely, advances have been made to help them thrive and survive. Advances in epidemiology have provided us with vaccines for a myriad of infectious diseases. All of these advancements have contributed (in one way or another) to a remarkable decrease in the infant mortality rate.

Many new instruments have made their way into the marketplace as well. **Ultrasound, magnetic resonance imaging** (MRI), and **computed axial tomography** (CAT) **scans** have made detecting injury or disease easier. Endoscopes have made treatment easier, requiring less down time, and lasers are proving useful in surgeries and other noninvasive procedures.

Medical skin care has become a more recent advancement. With a healthier and increasingly aged population, a premium has been placed on looking and feeling good. Improvements in how we care for our skin have made maintaining a younger look easier than it has ever been before.

MEDICAL TERMINOLOGY DEFINED

Just as teachers, auto mechanics, and computer engineers use words specific to their profession, so do medical personnel. As an aesthetician, you probably will not be using the word *megabyte* unless you are referring to

ultrasound
The use of sound waves to create an image.

magnetic resonance imaging
Noninvasive diagnostic technique that produces computerized images of internal body tissues and is based on nuclear magnetic resonance of atoms within the body that are induced by the application of radio waves.

computed axial tomography scans
A sectional view of the body shown by computed tomography.

someone who has a rather large mouth. If you were a computer analyst, you would use this term. Similarly, a virus will have a different meaning to you than it will to a computer analyst. The vocabulary you will be using is referred to as *medical terminology*.

As medical science grew and improved on itself, as new functions were understood, and as processes were discovered, the medical community adopted a language of its own, or vernacular. This vernacular was needed to help physicians and other allied health professionals keep straight the prolific amount of vocabulary involved in medicine.

How Medical Terminology Works

By knowing the meaning of Greek or Latin **root words,** the user can understand the meaning. The use of **suffixes** and **prefixes** gives further clarity. For example, you will learn that the meaning of the root *nephr* means pertaining to the kidneys. The suffix *ology* means the study of a subject. Therefore nephrology would be the study of the kidneys (Figure 2–7).

Medical terminology also includes the use of personal names as well. Usually, this use occurs in the context of a treatment or disorder that is named after the founder. For example, Dercum's disease, named for Francis X. Dercum, a U.S. neurologist.[1]

Why Use Medical Terminology?

By being consistent and learned in the area of medical terminology, you will be able to decipher the meaning of words, even if you have not heard the word. For example, if you are a specialist in the medical skin care area, you may encounter a word such as **dermatitis.** Although you may know

root words
Parts of Latin or Greek words that serve as the basis for medical terminology.

suffixes
Parts of Greek or Latin words used at the end of a word to alter or modify its meaning.

prefixes
Parts of Greek or Latin words used at the beginning of a word to alter or modify its meaning.

dermatitis
Inflammation of the skin.

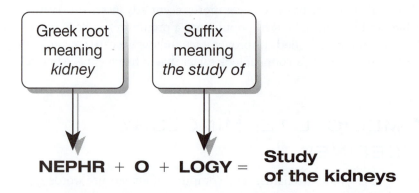

Figure 2–7   Diagrammatic breakdown of the word *nephrology*.

it is skin that itches or has a rash, the more interesting aspect would be that the exact meaning of dermatitis is skin inflammation.

HISTORY OF MEDICAL TERMINOLOGY

Way back when early physicians were first identifying anatomic structures, abnormalities, and functions, they realized a need to have an organized classification system. With so many words being added to the lexicon, setting in place a formalized, structured methodology for the naming process became necessary. Given that physicians were scattered across a wide geographic area and communication was slow and unreliable, early physicians needed to implement a system that would prevent things from being named multiple times, or named inconsistently. Try to imagine keeping track of the same item in several different languages. The father of medical terminology is the father of modern medicine himself, Hippocrates. Understanding how medical terminology has evolved over the centuries will help make sense of the vernacular in future chapters of this text.

Egyptian, Greek, and Roman Influences

To make order of the terminology to be used in medicine, Hippocrates was quite brilliant in his forethought in making the language of medicine universal. To accomplish this task, the father of modern medicine referred to the texts left behind by Imhotep, universally thought to be the father of medicine.

The knowledge that Imhotep passed on to his protégés was fine-tuned and adopted by the Romans. At the time, most Greek and Roman medical terms were based in mythology, legend, and physical description. Given that most of these myths and legends were meant to explain the unexplainable, the remnants of these words left in medical terminology are often amusing. For example, in Homer's myth, *The Odyssey*, drinking from the River Lethe leads to fatigue and sluggishness, or *lethargy*.[2]

Legends have also made permanent marks in the medical lexicon. The names Atlas, Achilles' heel, and cancer all have origins in legends of the day.[3]

Before the implementation of universal terminology, most terms were **coined** using physical descriptions. Kyphosis (hump back) is an example of this practice. The identification of disorders named for clinical descriptions was used routinely for the next few centuries.

coined
To create or invent a word or phrase.

Middle Ages and Renaissance Period

The coining of terms in the Middle Ages, as was the case with the Greeks and Romans, relied on clinical descriptions, even though they were often medically and politically incorrect. A term from this period is *clubfoot*. This disorder was so named because of the sound made on medieval castle floors.

As mentioned, a defining characteristic during the Renaissance was the increased intercontinental travel afforded by maritime advancements in shipbuilding and cartography. These advancements perpetuated a similar intercontinental influence in medical terminology. Cross-cultural hybrids of words began to appear. Words such as *orthopedics* come from the Latin word *ortho* (straight) and the Greek word *paedic (child).*

Contemporary Times

The medical community has organized to renovate prior mistakes and inaccuracies in nomenclature. Organizations and individuals have and are constantly searching for misnomers and other errors in the medical terminology. In many instances, several names for one item are retired, and one universally accepted name in accordance with the goals of medicine are accepted.

People who are seeking a career in medicine or the allied health fields today are schooled extensively on medical terminology and must use it when talking to their peers.

■ CONCLUSION

The history of medicine and medical technology goes hand in hand. As medical technology continues to expand on itself, the need for an organized and universal language for people in the medical profession becomes paramount. Learning about the history of medicine and how that overlaps with the creation of a universal lexicon will prove to be beneficial to all who study medical skin care.

▶▶▶ TOP 10 TIPS TO TAKE TO THE CLINIC

1. The history of medicine has much relevance to the procedures that the aesthetician performs.
2. Most of the medical advancements that we enjoy have their basis in earlier discoveries, but most were founded in the recent past.
3. The vernacular used in the allied health fields is called medical terminology.

4. Hippocrates began the process of identifying a universal language for people working in the medical fields.

5. Medical terminology employs the use of Greek and Latin root words, suffixes, and prefixes for words.

6. By knowing medical terminology, you will be able to decipher the meaning of words, even if you have not heard the word before.

7. Medical terminology also includes the use of personal names as well.

8. Medical terminology is constantly being added to and renovated to be more effective.

9. People who are seeking a career in medicine or the allied health fields today are schooled extensively on medical terminology and are encouraged to use it when talking to their peers.

10. You should always try to use medical terminology when talking to fellow health professionals.

CHAPTER REVIEW QUESTIONS

1. What are some of the early medical discoveries made by the Egyptians, the Greeks, and the Romans?
2. How are these discoveries pertinent to you as an aesthetician?
3. What medical advancements of the latter twentieth century have the most impact on your life? On your career as an aesthetician?
4. What is medical terminology?
5. Why is medical terminology necessary?
6. What are root words? Suffixes? Prefixes?
7. How have the ancients contributed to medical terminology?

CHAPTER 2 GLOSSARY OF KEY TERMS

Sir Alexander Fleming   Scottish physician and researcher who first discovered the ability of mold to kill bacteria.

antibiotics Class of drugs that kill bacteria.

bloodletting   Early medical treatment that used released blood from the body as a means of treating disease.

Claudius Galen   Protégé of Hippocrates who is credited with reviving and spreading his teachings.

coined   To create or invent a word or phrase.

computed axial tomography scans   Sectional view of the body shown by computed tomography.

deoxyribonucleic acid   Long, double strand of genetic information contained within cells; discovered by Wilkins, Crick, and Watt.

dermatitis   Inflammation of the skin.

Edward Jenner   British physician who discovered the vaccine for smallpox.

Hippocrates   Greek physician who is credited with being the father of modern medicine.

Sir Howard Walter Florey   Researcher who discovered penicillin.

Imhotep   First physician who lived in Egypt and was the pharaoh's personal physician around 2600 B.C.

Louis Pasteur   French scientist who discovered pasteurization.

magnetic resonance imaging   Noninvasive diagnostic technique that produces computerized images of internal body tissues.

medical terminology   Use of Greek and Latin roots, suffixes, and prefixes to denote diseases, conditions, and symptoms; used to create uniformity of language among medical professionals.

prefixes   Parts of Greek or Latin words used at the beginning of a word to alter or modify its meaning.

root words   Parts of Latin or Greek words that serve as the basis for medical terminology.

suffixes   Parts of Greek or Latin words used at the end of a word to alter or modify its meaning.

ultrasound   Use of sound waves to create an image.

CHAPTER REFERENCES

1. Thomas, C. L., (Ed.). (1997). *Taber's cyclopedic medical dictionary* (18th ed.). Philadelphia: F. A. Davis.
2. Bailey, J. A. (January 10, 2005). *The Black voice news* [Online]. Available: *http://www.blackvoices.com*.
3. Bailey, J. A. (January 10, 2005). *The Black voice news* [Online]. Available: *http://www.blackvoices.com*.

OTHER RESOURCES

Hubbard, K. (Feb. 7, 2005). *Everything you ever wanted to know about Proto-Indo-European (and the comparative method), but were afraid to ask!* [Online]. Available: *http://www.gen.umn.edu*.

Mosser, D. W. (Feb. 7, 2005). *The Evolution of Present-Day English.* [Online]. Available: *http://wiz.cath.vt.edu*.

Word Structure

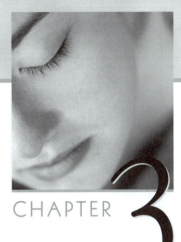

CHAPTER 3

KEY TERMS

adjective	diminutive	plural
combining form	modifies	pronunciation
combining vowel	noun	word analysis

LEARNING OBJECTIVES

After completing this chapter, you should be able to:

1. Isolate a root word through word analysis.

2. Identify a prefix through word analysis.

3. Identify a suffix through word analysis.

4. Combine root words with suffixes and prefixes to make new words.

5. Know how to make plurals.

6. Know how to pronounce words in medical terminology.

INTRODUCTION

Now that we have examined some of the broader fundamentals associated with medical terminology, you should be ready to begin the process of learning about the words themselves and some of the basics and exceptions that make medical terminology so complex.

As a patient, or student, you may have heard words that are easily recognizable and understood. For example, most people know what arthritis, tonsils, and kidneys are; but you may not know what a phlebotomist is or what laparoscopy is.

In this chapter, we learn to identify the various parts of the words and how to use them. The text is accompanied by exercises to help you better understand the concepts.

WORD ANALYSIS

word analysis

Process that separates the combined form of a word with the intention of ascertaining its meaning.

combining vowel

Vowel used to combine root words with suffixes and prefixes.

combining form

Resulting combination of a root word, a combining vowel, a prefix, a suffix, or any combination.

modifies

To qualify or limit the meaning of a word.

Medical terminology is similar to a puzzle. By using **word analysis** and dissecting a word, you can isolate the different parts of a word and unlock the puzzle. Once you can isolate the different parts of a word and define them, you can use this knowledge to help define many other pertinent words.

When examining a medical term, begin at the end of the word, or the suffix, and then go back to the beginning. For example, one word with which many people are familiar is *mammography*. The suffix of the word is *graphy,* which means *to record.* The root word here is *mamm,* which refers to the *breasts.* Therefore mammography is a recording of the breast.

To best find the suffix, isolate the different parts of the word. Look for the *o,* or another **combining vowel.** The root word and the combining vowel is the **combining form.** Here are some examples, beginning with the word *mammography:*

mammography	MAMM/O/GRAPHY
ophthalmoscope	OPHTHALM/O/SCOPE
pathology	PATH/O/LOGY
leukocyte	LEUK/O/CYTE
amniocentesis	AMNI/O/CENTESIS

In some instances, a medical term will have more than one root word. Given that the combining vowel connects the root word to the suffix, you will most often find a corresponding number of combining forms in this case.[1] Table 3–1 provides some examples. In many cases, a prefix will precede the combining form. A prefix **modifies** the root word, usually quantifying or qualifying it. For example, *poly* means *many,* and *intra* means *within.*

intravenous	INTRA/VEN/OUS
polyneuropathy	POLY/NEUR/O/PATHY

Let us look at some words in Table 3–2 and split them up accordingly. If you look at the examples in Table 3–2, you should note that not all words are structured in the exact same format. Notice that the word *intravenous* has no combining vowel. When the suffix, as is the case with *ous,* begins with a vowel, the combining vowel is dropped.

Table 3–1 Multiple Root Word Examples

Term	First Combining Form	Second Combining Form	Suffix
Gastroenterology	GASTRO	ENTERO	LOGY
Otolaryngologist	OTO	LARYNGO	LOGIST
Electroencephalography	ELECTRO	ENCEPHALO	GRAPHY

Table 3–2 Examples of Combining Vowel and Suffixes

Word	Prefix	Root Word	Combining Vowel	Suffix
Ophthalmoscope	N/A	OPHTHALM	O	SCOPE
Pathology	N/A	PATH	O	LOGY
Leukocyte	N/A	LEUK	O	CYTE
Amniocentesis	N/A	AMNI	O	CENTESIS
Intravenous	INTRA	VEN	N/A	OUS
Polyneuropathy	POLY	NEUR	O	PATHY

Some words have a prefix, others do not. The only thing that all words do have in common is the root word. To ascertain the meaning of a word, the most logical place to begin is with the root word.

ROOT WORDS

The root is the most basic component of a word, and it is the basis for which the meaning of a word is constructed. In many instances, roots can stand alone, as is the case with *graph, cycl(e), pyr(e), crypt,* and *term.* Most roots in medical terminology, however, do need other components. For example, the roots *gastr, carcin,* and *lapar* need to be combined with prefixes, suffixes, or even other roots.[2] Refer to Table 3–3 for examples.

A word can contain more than one root. For example, *matrilineal* contains the roots *matri* (mother) and *lineal* (line). Matrilineal therefore means *determining descent through the female line.*[5]

We will further explore root words in the following chapter.

Prefixes and suffixes change or modify a word's meaning. For example, the word *famous* means *well* or *widely known.*[3] With the prefix *in,* the word becomes *infamous,* which means *having an exceedingly bad reputation.*[4]

Table 3–3 Examples of Root Words

Root	Word	Definition
Gastr	Gastritis	Inflammation of the stomach
Carcin	Carcinogen	To produce cancer
Lapar	Laparotomy	Abdominal surgery

Table 3–4 Adjective Endings[6]

Adjective Endings	Example
-ac	cardiac (heart)
-al	skeletal (skeleton)
-ary	salivary (saliva)
-ic	pelvic (pelvis)
-ical	surgical (surgery)
-ous	venous (vein)
-tic	paralytic (paralysis)
-ar	muscular (muscle)

noun
Part of speech that is used to name a person, place, thing, quality or action. It is usually the subject or object of the action in a sentence.

adjective
Part of speech used to describe a noun.

plural
Form of a word meant to indicate that there is more than one.

diminutive
Suffix that is added to a word to note smallness or being smaller than something else.

SUFFIXES

Knowing the Greek and Latin origin of a word's suffix can help us determine the meaning. Prefixes modify their root words by indicating whether the word is a **noun, adjective, plural,** or **diminutive** (Tables 3–4, 3–5, and 3–6).

Suffixes help us determine the meaning of a word by describing the use of the word in question. The suffix tells us if the word is a noun or nouns, whether it describes something, or its relationship to something else.

PREFIXES

Knowing the Greek and Latin roots of a word's prefix can also help us determine the meaning of the word. As mentioned, prefixes modify the

Table 3–5 Noun Endings[7]

Noun Endings	Meaning	Example
-iac	Indicates a person afflicted with certain diseases or conditions	hemophiliac
-ia	An unhealthy state	anesthesia
-is	Forms the noun from the root	cutis (skin)
-ism	Condition, state of being	alcoholism (alcohol)
-ist	One who specializes	Dermatologist
-itis	Inflammation	arthritis
-logy	Study of	biology
-plasty	Form or fix	rhinoplasty
-oma	Tumor or mass	carcinoma
-scopy	Process of visual examination	laparoscopy
-y	Condition, process	neuropathy (nervous system disease)
-gen	To be produced	pathogen

Table 3–6 Diminutive Endings[8]

Diminutive Ending	Meaning	Example
-ole		arteriole (artery)
-icle	Small, little, minute	particle (piece)
-ule		venule (vein)

root words by either qualifying or quantifying them. Quantity can be determined by using the prefix *poly* to designate a general number or a specific number, as is the case with *tri*. Quantity can also be designated as a negation, such as *in* or *im,* meaning without.

Prefixes can also qualify the root in terms of temporal (meaning time) or directional. *Ante*, for instance, means *before;* and if we connect it with *mortem* which means death, we end up with *antemortem,* or before death. We will further explore prefixes later in this text.

Pneumonoultramicroscopicsilicovolcanokoniosis. Yes, this is an actual word. What does it mean? Medical terminology can be filled with words that sometimes seem incomprehensible. By *dissecting* these words into discrete units, even the most complex terms can be understood. By using these prefixes and suffixes, even the most difficult words such as this example can be easily understood.[9]

EXERCISES

Part A

Split up the following words as is shown in the example.

EXAMPLE: gastroscopy: GASTR/O/SCOPY

1. carcinogen _____

2. laparoscopy _____

3. adenoma _____

4. arthritis _____

5. biology _____

6. cephalic _____

7. cytology _____

8. electrocardiogram _____

9. enterology _____

10. hematoma _____

11. leukocyte _____

12. renal _____

13. pathogen _____

14. neural _____

15. psychosis _____

16. rhinoplasty _____

17. sarcoma _____

EXERCISES

Part B

Root Words: *Look up the definitions for each of the following root words.*

1. gastr _____

2. carcin _____

3. lapar _____

4. aden _____

5. athr _____

6. bi _____

7. cephal _____

8. cyt _____

9. electr _____

10. enter _____

11. hemat _____

12. leuk _____

13. ren _____

14. path _____

15. neur _____

16. psych _____

17. rhin _____

18. sarc _____

EXERCISES

Part C

Suffixes: *Define the following terms.*

1. gastric _____

2. carcinogen _____

3. laparoscopy _____

4. adenoma _____

5. arthritis _____

6. biology _____

7. cephalic _____

8. cytology _____

9. electrocardiogram _____

10. enterology _____

11. hematoma _____

12. leukocyte _____

13. renal _____

14. pathogen _____

15. neural _____

16. psychosis _____

17. rhinoplasty _____

18. sarcoma _____

■ PLURALS

As you know, the plural of many words in the English language are often difficult to ascertain. In some instances, the words are completely different (*mouse* and *mice*), or they are the same as the singular (*deer* and *deer*). A similar challenge exists for those of us in the medical communities. Some people might argue that the use of proper plurals can be one of the more challenging aspects of medical terminology. The problem is so pervasive that even many physicians experience difficulty with them.

Although difficult to understand, plurals generally follow some basic rules.[10] By taking the time to learn these rules, you will be prepared to tackle these challenges when they do arise. However, every rule has an exception. Nonetheless, exceptions are rare, as explained here.

The following table (Table 3–7) is meant to provide some of the more common rules of forming plurals.

Table 3–7 Basic Rules of Thumb for Forming Medical Plurals[11]

If the Singular Ending Is:	Singular Form	The Plural Rule Is:	Plural Form
-is	diagnosis	Drop the *is*, and add *es*	diagnoses
-um	ileum	Drop the *um*, and add *a*	ilea
-us	alveolus	Drop the *us*, and add *i*	alveoli
-a	vertebra	Drop the *a*, and add *ae*	vertebrae
-ix	appendix	Drop the *ix*, and add *ices*	appendices
-ex	cortex	Drop the *ex*, and add *ices*	Cortices
-ax	thorax	Drop the *x*, and add *ces*	Thoraces
-ma	sarcoma	Retain the *ma*, and add *ta*	Sarcomata
-on	spermatozoon	Drop the *on*, and add *a*	Spermatozoa
-nx	larynx	Drop the *x*, and add *ges*	Larynges
-y	deformity	Drop the *y*, and add *ies*	Deformities
-yx	calyx	Drop the *yx*, and add *yces*	Calyces
-en	foramen	Drop the *en*, and add *ina*	Foramina

Ten Common Exceptions to Basic Plural Rules[12]

1. In some words, the proper plural of a word ending in *is* will be formed by dropping the *is* and adding *ides*. For example, *epididymis* becomes *epididymides*.
2. In some words, the proper plural of a word ending in *us* will be formed by dropping the *us* and adding *era* or *ora*. For example, *viscus* becomes *viscera*; *corpus* becomes *corpora*.
3. Some words ending in *ix* or *ax* have more than one acceptable plural form. For example, the plural of *appendix* can be either *appendices* or *appendixes*, although the most common plural form would use the *ices* ending.
4. The proper plural for certain words ending in *ion* can be formed simply by adding an *s*. For example, *chorion* becomes *chorions*.
5. The plural form of the term *vas* is *vasa*.
6. The plural form of *pons* is *pontes*.
7. The plural form of the dual meaning word *os* is *ora* when referring to *mouths* and *ossa* when referring to *bones*.
8. The plural form of the term *femur* is *femora*.
9. The plural form of *cornu* is *cornua*.
10. The plural form of *paries* is *parietes*.

EXERCISES

Part D

Write in the corresponding singular endings for the following plural endings:

1. -ae   _____

2. -ces   _____

3. -ina   _____

4. -ices _____

5. -ses   _____

6. -a   _____

7. -i   _____

8. -ies   _____

9. -mata _____

EXERCISES

Part E

Write in the plurals to the singular words in the space provided:

1. index _____   6. patella _____

2. thorax _____   7. ovum _____

3. deformity _____   8. lumen _____

4. ganglion _____   9. diagnosis _____

5. carcinoma _____

PRONUNCIATION

Pronunciation is a fundamental yet key concept for anyone in the allied medical fields. Regardless of the vast wealth of knowledge a brain may contain, viewing a person as credible will be difficult unless he or she pronounces the vernacular with precision. In medical terminology, many words are long and complicated, and they are thus rather easy to mispronounce. For anyone who intends to work with patients or other medical personnel, he or she must have a grasp on pronunciation. Having accurate pronunciation skills will require both patience and diligence.

Words that have the following combination of letters at the beginning of the word are often said in the following way (Table 3–8):

pronunciation
Process of accurately speaking a word as it is meant to be spoken.

Table 3–8 Silent Letters[13]

Letter Combination	Sound	Example	Pronunciation
pt	t	pterygoid	ter'-ĭ-gold
ps	s	psoriasis	sor-i'-ah-sis
pn	n	pneometer	ne-om'-it-er
gn	n	gnathitis	na-thĭt'-is
mn	n	mnemonic	ne-mon'-ik

If a prefix ending in a vowel comes before the following combination of letters, then the first letter is pronounced:

hemoptysis	he-mop'-tî-sis
prognathism	prog'-nah-tizm
polypnea	pol"-ip-ne'-ah
dysgnathia	dis-na'-the-ah

Combination of vowels—*oe* and *ae* (English spelling)—are pronounced as *ee; ce, cae,* and *coe* as *see* and *ge, gae,* and *goe* as *jee* in English.

haema	he'-mah
rugae	roo'-je
coelum	se'-lom
septicaemia	sep"-tî-se'-me-ah
caecum	se'-kum

Another combination of letters is pronounced in the following way (Table 3–9)[14]:

Table 3–9 Letter-Specific Pronunciations

Letter Combination	Sound	Word	Pronunciation
ph	f	phrenoplegia	fren"-o-ple'-je-ah
rh	r	rhytidosis	rit"-î-do'-sis
ch	k	cochlea	kok'-le-ah
x	z	xanthic	zan'-thik
dys	dis	dysphagia	dis-fa'-je-ah

EXERCISES

Pronunciation

Write out the correct spelling for the phonetic pronunciation in brackets:

1. [dis-fa'-je-ah] _____

2. [prog'-nah-tizm] _____

3. [fren"-o-ple'-je-ah] _____

4. [kok'-le-ah] _____

EXERCISES

Pronunciation—cont'd

Write out the correct spelling for the phonetic pronunciation in brackets:

5. [he-mop'-tî-sis]   _____

6. [pol"-ip-ne'-ah]   _____

7. [na-thît'-is]   _____

8. [dis-na'-the-ah]   _____

9. [ne-mon'-ik]   _____

10. [he'-mah]   _____

11. [ne-om'-it-er]   _____

12. [roo'-je]   _____

13. [rit"-î-do'-sis]   _____

14. [se'-lom]   _____

15. [sor-i'-ah-sis]   _____

16. [sep"-tî-se'-me-ah]   _____

17. [ter'-î-gold]   _____

18. [zan'-thik]   _____

CONCLUSION

We have now advanced from the history of the English language and the history of medical terminology to the core fundamentals of word analysis and dissection. We have discussed the different components of a word and how to isolate them. Taking this information a step further, we have learned how to pluralize and pronounce them as well. Together, these concepts comprise the fundamentals of medical terminology. Moving forward, we will narrow our scope and examine some of the same topics discussed herein while broadening your scope of comprehension on medical terminology.

TOP 10 TIPS TO TAKE TO THE CLINIC

1. Once you can isolate the different parts of a word and define them, you can use this knowledge to help define many other pertinent words.

2. The root is the most basic component of a word, and it is the basis for which the meaning of a word is constructed.

3. When examining a medical term, begin at the end of the word and then go back to the beginning.

4. Look for the *o* or another combining vowel. The root word and the combining vowel is the combining form.

5. In some instances, a medical term will have more than one root word. Given that the combining vowel connects the root word to the suffix, you will most often find a corresponding number of combining forms in this case.

6. In many words, a prefix will be placed before the combining form. A prefix modifies the root word, usually quantifying or qualifying it.

7. Knowing the Greek and Latin origin of a word's suffix can help us determine the meaning.

8. Some people might argue that the use of proper plurals can be one of the more challenging aspects of medical terminology.

9. Knowing the Greek and Latin roots of a word's prefix can also help us determine the meaning of words.

10. Having accurate pronunciation skills will require both patience and diligence.

CHAPTER REVIEW QUESTIONS

1. How should you dissect a word to decipher its meaning?
2. What is a combining vowel?
3. What is a combining form?
4. What is a prefix? What does it do? Where is it?
5. What is a root word? Why is it important?
6. What is a suffix? Where is a suffix in a word?
7. What is the plural of vertebra? What is the plural for diagnosis?
8. What do the letter combinations *gn, pt,* and *ps* all have in common in medical terminology?

CHAPTER 3 GLOSSARY OF KEY TERMS

adjective   Part of speech used describe a noun.
combining vowel   Vowel used to combine root words with suffixes and prefixes.
combining form   Resulting combination of a root word, a combining vowel, a prefix, a suffix, or any combination.
diminutive   Suffix that is added to a word to note smallness or being smaller than something else.

modifies   To qualify or limit the meaning of a word.

noun   Part of speech that is used to name a person, place, thing, quality or action. It is usually the subject or object of the action in a sentence.

plural   Form of a word meant to indicate that there is more than one.

pronunciation   Process of accurately speaking a word as it is meant to be spoken.

word analysis   Process of separating the combined form of a word with the intention of ascertaining its meaning.

CHAPTER REFERENCES

1. Chabner, D-E. (2003). *Medical terminology: A short course* (3rd ed.). Philadelphia, PA: W. B. Saunders.
2. Dummies.com. (Feb. 16, 2005). *Tending to word roots (adapted from vocabulary for dummies)* [Online]. Available: *http://www.dummies.com*
3. Dictionary.com. (Feb. 15, 2005). *Word search: Famous* [Online]. Available: *http://dictionary.reference.com*
4. Dictionary.com. (Feb. 15, 2005). *Word search: Famous* [Online]. Available: *http://dictionary.reference.com*
5. Dummies.com. (Feb. 16, 2005). *Tending to word roots (adapted from vocabulary for dummies)* [Online]. Available: *http://dictionary.reference.com*
6. Cohen, B. J. (1998). *Medical terminology: An illustrated guide.* Philadelphia, PA: Lippincott-Raven Publishers.
7. Cohen, B. J. (1998). *Medical terminology: An illustrated guide.* Philadelphia, PA: Lippincott-Raven Publishers.
8. Cohen, B. J. (1998). *Medical terminology: An illustrated guide.* Philadelphia, PA: Lippincott-Raven Publishers.
9. About.com. (Feb 16, 2005). Biology: *Bio-word dissection* [Online]. Available: *http://biology.about.com*
10. MTWorld.com. (Feb 12, 2005). *Forming plurals of medical words* [Online]. Available: *http://mtworld.com*
11. MTWorld.com. (Feb 12, 2005). *Forming plurals of medical words* [Online]. Available: *http://mtworld.com*
12. MTWorld.com. (Feb 12, 2005). *Forming plurals of medical words* [Online]. Available: *http://mtworld.com*
13. Gyls, B. A., & Wedding, M. E. (1983). *Medical terminology: A systems approach.* Philadelphia, PA: F. A. Davis.
14. Gyls, B. A., & Wedding, M. E. (1983). *Medical terminology: A systems approach.* Philadelphia, PA: F. A. Davis.

Root Words

CHAPTER 4

LEARNING OBJECTIVES

After completing this chapter, you should be able to:

1. Recognize a root word as having a Greek or Latin origin.
2. Learn the most common Greek roots.
3. Learn the most common Latin roots.
4. Complete exercises designed to enhance your understanding of root words.

INTRODUCTION

By this point, you should be able to dissect a word using word analysis. However, as you may know, dissecting a word and interpreting its meaning are two different stories. In this chapter, we will be delving into the content that comprises the crux of medical terminology. As we mentioned, the roots of words form the basis for a word's meaning. In this chapter, we will explore the Greek and Latin roots that make up the majority of medical terminology. To aid in your understanding, exercises will be provided, and their usage is encouraged.

ROOT WORD BASICS

All words have a root.* The root of a word will provide the clues you need to reveal the meaning. For example, the root of *becoming* is *come*. Given that we know what *come* means (a form of *to be*), we have the first clue needed to encode the meaning. In another example, let us use the word *misogynist*. If we dissect this word using word analysis, it appears in the following way:

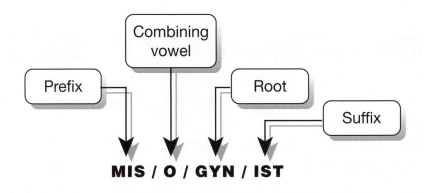

In this chapter, we will take this analysis to the next level. Being able to dissect the word is one thing, knowing what the individual parts are is another, but knowing what those individual parts mean is still another.

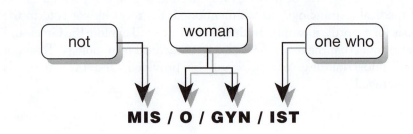

---

* Soltesz-Steiner, S. (2003). *Quick medical terminology: A self-teaching guide.* Hoboken, NJ: John Wiley & Sons.

Words with the same root will have related meanings, as shown in the following example:

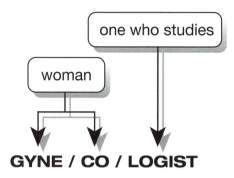

The next few chapters are intended to help you achieve this level of interpretation.

Part A

Find the root word in each of the following words:

1. import/export _____

2. decision/indecision _____

3. dictate/dictaphone _____

4. prognosis/prognosticate _____

5. encephalitis/encephalopathy _____

6. indicative/ridiculous _____

7. airport/portal _____

GREEK ROOT WORDS A TO Z

In this section, we will identify the more common root words that have their origins in Greek. The Greek roots are listed alphabetically followed by their meaning and examples. Exercises will follow.

ACANTH (thorn)

acantholysis Skin disease characterized by the atrophy of the prickle cell layer
acanthosis Benign growth of the prickle cell layer

ACR (extremity)

acropodium Finger or toe tips

ACTIN (ray)

actinic Specific to the rays on the spectrum that are capable of producing chemical change

ADEN (gland)

heteradenia Abnormal formation of a gland
adenopathy Any disease of the glands

AER (gas or air)

aeropathy Any disorder caused by a change in pressure
anaerobic Not requiring air or oxygen to sustain life

ALG (pain)

analgesic Remedy for relieving pain
neuralgia Nerve pain
causalgia Burning type of pain
arthralgia Joint pain

ALL (different)

allogamy Cross-fertilization
allergy Hypersensitive state

ANCON (elbow)

anconitis Inflammation of the elbow

ANDR (male)

andromorphous Having the shape or structure of man

ANGI (vessel)

angiitis Inflammation of the blood vessels

ANTH (flower)

exanthema Eruption outside the body, or on the skin

ARTHR (joint, speech)

arthritis Inflammation of the joints
dysarthria Speech impairment
enarthrosis Any ball-and-socket type of joint, as in the shoulder

diarthrosis Freely movable articulation
nearthrosis Disorder characterized by abnormal articulation in a bone
arthralgia Joint pain

ANTHROP (human being)

anthropophilic Preferring humans over other animals

ANTR (cavity)

antritis Inflammation of the sinus cavity

AUT (self)

autism Inward concentration on oneself
autophagia Psychologic disorder characterized by biting one's own flesh

AUX (to increase)

onychauxis Hypertrophy of the nail

BA (to walk)

basophobia Fear of walking

BALL, BOL (to throw or to place)

metabolism Breakdown of food substances into energy
embolism Obstruction of a blood vessel by lodging a foreign material in it
anabolism Synthetic metabolism

BI (life)

biomorphic Related to the living form
symbiosis Union of two organisms for mutual benefit
biopsy Examination of living tissue
biotherapy Treatment of disease with substances found in nature
metabiosis Relationship between two organisms in which one benefits (e.g., a black widow spider kills her mate after seeding her eggs)
psychobiology Psychology in relation to biology
antibiotic Relationship between two organisms in which one will kill the other

BLAST (seed or bud)

lipoblast Formative fat cell

BLEPHAR (eyelid)

blepharoplasty Cosmetic or corrective surgery on the eyelid

BOL, BOUL (will)

hyperboulia Exaggerated willfulness
dysbulia Inability to harness willpower

BRACHY (short)

brachypodous Short footed

BRADY (slow)

bradycardia Abnormally slow heartbeat
bradylexia Abnormally slow at reading

BROM (foul scent, bromine)

bromoderma Eruptions on the skin caused by ingestion of bromine

BRONCH, BRONCHI (airway)

bronchitis Inflammation of bronchial tubes
bronchocele Bronchial dilation

CARCIN (cancer)

carcinogen Any substance known or thought to cause cancer
carcinoma Malignant growth

CARDI (pertaining to the heart)

diplocardiac Having two hearts or a heart wherein the two sides are separate
myocardial Pertaining to the muscular tissue of the heart
exocardial Occurring outside the heart

CARP (wrist)

metacarpal Part of the hand between the wrist and the digits

CAU (to burn)

cauterize To burn tissue using an agent or instrument

CELE (hernia or swelling)

enterocele Hernia that involves a loop of the intestines
hydrocele Buildup of fluid in the testicles
hydromyelocele Accumulation of fluid in the spinal cord
myelocele Spina bifida with a protrusion of the spinal cord

CENTE (to puncture)

enterocentesis Surgical puncture of the intestines
pneumonocentesis Surgical puncture of the lungs

CEPHAL (head)

acrocephaly Deformity characterized by an abnormally pointed head

CHEIL, CHIL (lip)

acheilia Congenital absence of the lips
cheiloplasty Corrective or plastic surgery on the lips

CHIR (hand)

chiroplasty Any cosmetic or corrective surgery on the hands

CHOL (bile)

cholochrome Any pigment in bile
eucholia Normal state of bile

CHORD (cord)

chorditis Inflammation of the spermatic cord
iridochoroiditis Inflammation of the choroids and the iris

CHROM, CHROMAT (color)

chromatin Photosensitive substance within the cells that change color

CHRON (time)

heterochronism Deviation in the normal time sequence for a given process

CLAS (break)

cardioclasis Rupture in the tissue of the heart

CLY (to wash or to rinse)

hypodermoclysis Use of large quantities of fluid into subcutaneous tissues
phleboclysis To flush a vein using saline

COCC (berrylike)

Streptococcus Chain-forming bacteria

COL (colon)

coloproctostomy Surgical creation of a new passage from the colon to the rectum

COLL, COLLA (glue)

collagen Protein found in connective tissue

CONDYL (knob)

condyle Rounded protrusion such as those at the end of bones
condyloma Tumor resembling a wart

CRANI (cranium)

amphicrania Headache affecting both sides of the head
pericranium Outer surface of the cranial bones

CRINE (to secrete)

endocrine Excreted internally
exocrine Excreted externally
neurocrine Secretion from newer cells

CRY, CRYM (cold)

cryesthesia Sensitivity to cold

CRYPT (hidden)

cryptorchism Condition in which the male gonads fail to drop
cryptogenic Of unknown origin or cause

CYCL (circle)

acyclia Cessation of body fluid circulation

CYE (to be pregnant)

cyophoria Gestation

CYST (bladder, cyst)

cystitis Inflammation of the bladder
hematocyst Blood-filled cyst
polycystic Many cysts

CYT (cell)

chromocyte Any cell with pigmentation
cytolysis Destruction of cells

DACTYL (finger or digit)

orthodactylous Having straight digits
oxydactyl Slender or tapered digits
syndactylism Webbed or fused fingers or toes

DEM (people)

pandemic Disease occurring over a wide geographic area affecting many people
endemic Disease that is confined to a particular locale

DERM, DERMAT (skin)

dermatophyte Group of fungi that resides underneath the skin and appendages
dermographia Condition in which the skin is particularly susceptible to irritation
mesoderm Layer of skin that houses connective tissue and muscles

DESM (ligaments)

syndesmology Study of ligaments

DIDYM (twin or testicle)

anandidymus Substandard duplicity

DROM (course)

syndrome Sequence of symptoms that collectively characterize a disease

heterodromia Condition in which a nerve's impulses are stronger in one of two directions

DYN, DYNAM (power)

hemodynamics Study of blood, circulation, and blood pressure

EC, EK, OIC, OIK (house)

ecology Study of animals and how they interact with their environment

ECH (to repeat)

echolalia Repetition of words without cohesion

echocardiogram Test using sound waves to create an image of the heart for use as diagnostic tool

echoencephalogram Test using of sound waves to create an image of the brain for use as diagnostic tool

EDE (to swell)

edema Swelling caused by fluid accumulation within tissue

EO (dawn or red)

Eolithic Earliest period of the stone age

ERG (to work)

hypergia Increase in functional activity

hyperergy Sensitivity to allergens

ERYTHR (red)

erythrodermia Condition characterized by redness of the skin

ESTHE, AESTHE (to feel)

akinesthesia Loss of mobile sensitivity

GALA, GALACT (milk)

galactin Hormone that stimulates lactation

GAM (union)

gamete Sex cell

autogamy Self-fertilization

oogamy Union of the female egg and the male sperm

GE (earth)

amphigean Native to all parts of the world

GER, GERONT (old age)

gerontophobia Extreme fear of aging

progeria Premature senility

GLAUC (silver or gray)

glaucoma Eye disease characterized by heightened intraocular tension

GLOT (tongue)

epiglottis Membrane that protects the glottis while swallowing

GLYC (sugar)

glycolysis Conversion of carbohydrates into lactic or pyruvic acid

hyperglycemia Excess sugar in the bloodstream

GNO (to know or have knowledge)

asterognosis Inability to recognize things by touch

prognosis Educated guess as to cause, course, and treatment of a given set of symptoms

GON (to produce)

gonad Sex gland (testes or ovaries)

GONI (angle)

gonimeter Instrument used to measure angles

HELI (sun)

heliotaxis Response to the stimulus of
  sunlight

HEM, HEMAT (blood)

haematobic Living in the blood
hematocrit Centrifuge used to separate blood
  cells
hemolytic Destruction of red blood cells

HEPAT, HEPAR (liver)

heparin Substance in the liver that can prolong
  blood clotting

HETER (different)

heterokinesis Movement caused by external
  stimuli
heterosexual Person who has sex with members
  of the opposite sex

HIST, HISTI (tissue)

histokinesis Activity of the smallest known
  structures of the body

HOD, OD (road or path)

anode Positive electrode
esodic Afferent nerve sending signals to the
  central nervous system

HYAL (glass)

hyaline Clear material found in bodily colloids
  and jellies
hyaloid Clear or glasslike

HYDR (fluid)

hydrarthrosis Fluid accumulation in a joint
hydrotropism Response of a subject to water

HYGR (moisture)

hygrokinesis Movement in response to moisture
  or humidity
hygrostomia Chronic salivation

HYSTER (uterus)

hysterotomy Caesarian section
hysterectomy Removal of the uterus

IS (same)

isometric Equal in measure

ISCH (to suppress)

ischesis Reabsorption of a discharge
ischemia Localized reduction of blood flow
  caused by obstruction
ischuria Retention of urine

ISCHI (hip)

ischiodidymus Conjoined twins joined at the hip

KER, KERAT (horny tissue)

keratinization Development of horny tissue

KINE (motion)

kinesiology Science of anatomy and physiology
telekinesis Ability to move an object without
  touching it

LAL (to talk)

heterolalia To say one thing when another is meant

LAPAR (abdomen)

laparotomy Any surgery involving an incision
  into the abdomen

LARYNG (larynx)

otolaryngology Field of medicine that emphasizes
  the ears, nose, and throat

LECITH (yolk)

lectin Waxy material distributed through the
  body and in egg yolks

LEI (smooth)

leiodermia Condition characterized by abnormal
  glossiness of the skin

LEP (to seize)

narcolepsy Condition characterized by sudden fits of deep sleep (i.e., hypnolepsy)

epilepsy Condition characterized by sudden seizures

LEPT (delicate)

leptodermatous Thin skinned

LEX (to read)

bradylexia Abnormal slowness in reading

dyslexia Disorder that results in complications in reading or writing

LIP (fat)

lipodystrophy Condition characterized by the elimination of fat in certain parts of the body but not other parts

lipolysis Destruction of fat and fat cells

LOG (word)

dyslogia Difficulty articulating thoughts

LYMPH (pertaining to the lymph glands)

lymphoderma Condition affecting the lymphatics of the skin

MACR (large)

macrogamy Reproduction between two full-grown members of a given species

macroscopic Large enough to be seen by the unaided eye

MAST, MAZ (breast)

acromastitis Inflammation of the nipple

hypermastia Overgrowth of the mammary gland

mastectomy Removal of the breast

MEGA (large)

megalomania High opinion of oneself

MEL (limbs)

amelus Person missing a limb or limbs

MELAN (dark)

melanin Dark-brown pigment

melanism Abnormal pigmentation of tissue

melanoderma Dark, mispigmentation of the skin

MEN (moon, menstruation)

menarche First menstrual period

menopause Secession of the menstrual cycle

MENING (membrane)

meningitis Inflammation of the membranes of the spinal cord

MER (part)

myomere Segment of muscle

MES (middle)

mesomorphic Having a muscular, athletic build

mesophlebitis Middle coat of a vein

MICR (small)

micromelia Abnormally small limbs

MIS (hate)

misanthropy Hatred of mankind

MIT (thread)

mitosis Indirect cell division

mitochondria Cytoplasmic organelles within the cells

MNE (to remember)

amnesia Long-term memory loss

pseudomnesia False memories

mnemodermia Pruritus and pain of the skin after eliminating the symptoms

MORPH (to form or to change)

morphology Study of structure and form

dysmorphophobia Fear of deformation

anaorphosis Gradual evolution from one to another

MY, MYO, MYOS (muscle)

myochrome Muscle pigment

MYEL (spinal cord)

myelin White sheath protecting some nerves

MYX (mucus)

myxasthenia Inability to secrete mucus

NARC (stupor)

narcotic Drug that causes a state of motor or sensory impairment

NE (new)

nearthrosis Bone disorder characterized by abnormal articulation
neanthropic Same species as recent man
neoplasm Any new growth

NECR (dead tissue)

necrosis Pertaining to dead tissue

NEPHYR (kidney)

perinephrium Connective tissue of the kidney

NEUR (nerve, nervous system)

neuroanatomy The nervous system
neurotomy Division of a nerve

NOS (disease)

nosogeography Geography of disease

ODONT (tooth)

exodontist Dentist who specializes in tooth extraction
prosthodontia Sect of dentistry that specializes in artificial tooth replacement

ODYN (pain)

myodynia Muscle pain
odynophobia Fear of being in pain

OLIG (few)

oligotrichia Thinning of the hair

ONC, ONCUS (tumor)

adenoncus Glandular tumor

OO (egg)

ooblastoma Egg after fertilization
oocye Egg before the creation of the first polar body

OP, OPT (eye)

myopia Nearsighted
optician Person who makes corrective eyewear

OPTHALM (pertaining to the eye)

xerophthalmia Condition in which the conjunctiva is dry and hardened
exophthalmic Abnormal protrusion of the eyeball from its socket
ophthalmologist Person who specializes in the treatment of disorders affecting the eye

ORCH (testicle)

cryptorchism Condition in which the male gonads fail to drop

ORTH (straight)

orthoptic Normal binocular vision

OSM (sense of smell)

anosmia Inability to smell

OST (bone)

hetero-osteoplasty Grafting of a bone, using the bone of another animal
osteomyelitis Inflammation of the bone marrow

OT (ear)

diotic Affecting both ears
parotid Situated near the ear

OX, OXY (sharp; oxygen)

oxydactyl Having long, pointed digits

PAG (united)

craniopagus Conjoined twins joined at the head
hypogastropagus Conjoined twins joined in the stomach region

PALI (return)

palindromia Relapse

PAN (all)

pandemic Disease occurring over a wide geographic area affecting many people

PATH (disease or feeling)

idiopathic Disease for which no known cause has been discovered
pathology Study of disease

PED, PAED (child)

orthopedic Pertaining to the branch of surgery devoted to the correction of locomotive deformities, formerly devoted to correction of deformities in children
pediatrics Pertaining to the study of childhood disease

PEN (deficiency)

glycopenia Tendency toward hypoglycemia

PEP, PEPT (to digest)

peptic Pertaining to digestion

PETR (rock)

osteopetrosis Abnormally increased bone density

PHA (to speak)

schizophasia Scrambled words that usually occur in conjunction with schizophrenia
aphasia Loss of the ability to use words

PHAG (to eat)

autophagia Psychologic disorder characterized by biting one's own flesh
dysphagia Disorder characterized by a difficulty swallowing
phagocyte Unattached cell that ingests foreign matter

PHALAC(T) (to guard or protect)

exophylaxis Protection by skin secretions against pathogenic agents
anaphylactic State of super sensitivity after exposure to an antigen

PHAN (to appear)

menophania First appearance of menses

PHLEB (vein)

phlebismus Swelling of a vein
phleboclysis Process of flushing a vein using saline

PHON (sound)

dysphonia Voice impairment

PHOR, PHER (to bear, to go)

oophorectomy Surgical removal of an ovary
euphoria Exaggerated state of happiness
chromatophore Pigment-loaded cell
diaphoresis Noticeably abundant perspiration

PHOT (light)

photolytic Able to be decomposed with light

PHRAG (to contain within)

emphractic Having the quality of blocking the excretory functions of the skin

PHRAS (to speak)

aphrasia Inability to speak articulately

PHREN (mind)

phrenic Pertaining to the mind
hypophrenia Having or relating to feeblemindedness

PHY (to grow)

apophysis Projection of an organ

PHYLL (leaf)

phyllopodous Having leaflike feet

PHYTE (plant or growth)

autophyte Self-nourishing plant
hematophyte Plant or vegetative organism living in the blood

PLAS, PLAST (to form or mold)

hyperplasia Excessive tissue formation caused by increased cell production
rhinoplasty Plastic surgery done to reshape the tissue in or around the nose

PLATY, PLATYS (broad)

platysma Subcutaneous muscle in the neck

PLEG (paralysis)

paraplegia Paralysis of the lower limbs
laryngoplegia Paralysis of the larynx
quadriplegia Paralysis of all four limbs

PLEUR (side)

anisopleural Bilaterally asymmetrical

PLEX (stroke)

apoplexy Complex resulting from hemorrhaging from or onto the brain
cataplexy Sudden muscular rigidity produced by fear in some animals

PLO (fold)

diplopia Double vision

PNEA (breathing)

hyperpnea Breathing that is more rapid compared with normal respiration

PNEUM (air)

pneumatization Having air-filled cavities in the bones

POD, PUS (foot)

podiatrist Person who treats foot disorders
micropus Abnormally small feet

POIKIL (irregular)

poikiloderma Irregular skin pigmentation
poikilodermatomyositis Poikiloderma, usually concurrent with muscular sclerosis

POLY (many)

polyphagia Eating various kinds of food
polypod Having many feet or legs
polyuria Passage of excessive amounts of urine

POR (passageway)

digonoporous Male and female genital apertures

PRESBY (old)

presbyatrics Field of study dealing with the diseases associated with old age

PROCT (anus or rectum)

proctology Medical specialty emphasizing the study of the anus, rectum, and colon
proctostasis Constipation caused be a nonresponsive rectum

PSEUD (false or fake)

chromatopseudopsis Color blindness
pseudocyst Saclike space containing liquid

PSYCH (mind)

psyche The mind as the collective association between the mind, the soul, and free will and how they all interact with the world around us

psychopathic Behaving in a manner that is inconsistent with what is considered appropriate

PTO (to fall)

proptosis Prolapse

PY (pus)

pyorrhea Puslike discharge

pyuria Pus in the urine

PYL (gateway)

pylethrombophlebitis Inflammation with thrombosis of the portal vein

PYR, PYRE (heat or fire)

pyretolysis Fever reduction

RHIN, RHINE (nose)

rhinoplasty Plastic surgery done to reshape the tissue in or around the nose

SARC (flesh)

sarcobiont Living on skin

sarcoma Malignant tumor on connective tissues

SCHIZ, SCHIS (to split)

schistocyte Part of a red blood cell containing hemoglobin

schizophrenic Mental condition characterized by hearing voices or split personalities, or both

SCLER (hardened)

sclera Fibrous outer coating of the eyeball

SCOP (to view)

cryoscope Device used to freeze liquids

endoscope Instrument used to view the inside of the body through a natural orifice

SEP (to rot)

antiseptic Ability to destroy microorganisms that cause sepsis

aseptic Condition characterized by being free from germs

septic Condition characterized by being infected by germs

SOM, SOMAT (body)

dermatosome Vital component of the cell membrane

meromicrosomia Abnormal smallness of a body part

SPA (to jerk)

spasmophilia Predisposition toward convulsions

SPHYGM (pulse)

sphygmograph Instrument used to measure the variations in pulse

STA (to stand)

orthostatic Caused from standing upright

STAPHYL (bunches)

Staphylococcus Bacteria with the tendency to appear in clusters

STEN (narrow)

stenostomatous Having a narrow mouth

STERN (chest)

chondrosternal Pertaining to the chest and surrounding areas

sternum Connective tissue that joins the ribs at the chest

STIG (mark or point)

astigmatism Abnormal curvature of refractive surfaces within the eye, resulting in poor vision

STOL, STAL, STLE (to send, to contract)

systole Contraction of the heart

anastalsis Antiperistalsis

catastalsis Downward movement of stomach muscles during digestion

hemisystole Left ventricular contraction after every other atrial contraction

diastole Rhythmic relaxation stage of the heartbeat

bradydiastolic Prolonged diastolic interval

STOM, STOMAT (mouth or opening)

stomatitis Inflammation of the mouth

anastomosis Intercommunication of blood vessels with regard to blood pathways

SYRING (tube)

syringe Instrument used to inject agents into the body

TACHY (fast)

tachycardia Excessively rapid heartbeat

TAX (to arrange)

phototaxis Response to a light stimulus

TELO (completion)

atelopodia Defects in the development of the foot

THE (to put)

allenthesis Introduction of foreign matter into the body

prosthetic Artificial part that replaces one that is lost or missing

THEL (nipple)

endothelium Lining of blood vessels

epithelium Tissue that forms the epidermis

mesothelium Tissue lining the body cavity

THERM (heat)

hyperthermalgesia Sensitivity to heat

hypothermia Dangerously low body temperature

THORAC (chest)

hemothorax Accumulation of blood in the chest cavity

THROM (clot)

thrombocyte Blood platelet

TON (tension)

tonus Normal muscle state characterized by partial contraction

TOP (to place)

topical To place externally

TOX (poison)

cytotoxin Cell-poisoning substance found in blood serum

toxidermatitis Skin inflammation as a result of poisoning

antitoxin Any substance that can counteract the effects of poisoning

toxicology Study of poisons and their effects on the body

TRACHEL (neck)

laparotrachelotomy Low cesarean section through the neck of the uterus

TRICH (hair)

melanotrichous Dark haired

TROP, TREP (to turn or to respond accordingly)

phototropic Response to light stimulus

esotropia Condition of the eye in which one eye drifts inward

orthotropism Growth in a vertical line

TROPH (development)

autotroph Capable of self-nourishment
hypertrophy Size increase independent of normal growth
dystrophy Inadequate or compromised nutrition

UR, URE (having to do with urine or urination)

ureter Pathway for urine from the kidney to the bladder
uremic Presence of urine in the blood
albuminuria Presence of albumin in the urine
diuretic Agent that increases urine volume

XEN (stranger)

xenophobia Fear of leaving a place of safety, usually one's home

XER (dry)

xeroderma Dry skin

ZYM (to ferment)

zymosis Fermentation

EXERCISES

Part B

Match the word from the list of definitions.

_____ 1. quadriplegia
_____ 2. xeroderma
_____ 3. toxicology
_____ 4. diuretic
_____ 5. hypertrophy
_____ 6. topical
_____ 7. thrombocyte
_____ 8. epithelium
_____ 9. mesothelium
_____ 10. melanotrichous
_____ 11. staphylococcus
_____ 12. orthostatic
_____ 13. dermatosome
_____ 14. pseudocyst
_____ 15. septic
_____ 16. sclera
_____ 17. poikiloderma
_____ 18. platysma
_____ 19. aphrasia
_____ 20. syringe

a. Not requiring air or oxygen to sustain life
b. Dry skin
c. Agent that increases urine volume
d. Dark haired
e. Study of poisons and their effects on the body
f. To place externally
g. Test using sound waves to create an image of the heart for use as a diagnostic tool
h. Tissue that forms the epidermis
i. Instrument used to inject agents into the body
j. Bacteria with the tendency to appear in clusters
k. Caused from standing upright
l. Fibrous outer coating of the eyeball
m. Subcutaneous muscle in the neck
n. Psychologic disorder characterized by biting one's own flesh
o. Vital component of the cell membrane
p. Irregular skin pigmentation
q. Inability to speak articulately
r. Paralysis of all four limbs
s. Size increase independent of normal growth
t. Blood platelet
u. Tissue lining the body cavity
v. Saclike space containing liquid
w. Condition characterized as being infected by germs

EXERCISES

Part C

Match the following root words with the body parts that define their meaning.

1. ACR _____

2. ADEN _____

3. ANCON _____

4. ANTR _____

5. ARTHR _____

6. BLEPHAR _____

7. BRONCH _____

8. CARDI _____

9. CARP _____

10. CEPAHAL _____

11. CHEIL _____

12. CHIR _____

13. COL _____

14. CRANI _____

15. CYST _____

16. CYT _____

17. DACTYL _____

18. DERM _____

19. DESM _____

20. DIDYM _____

21. GLOT _____

22. HEMAT _____

23. HEPAT _____

24. HIST _____

25. HYSTER _____

26. ISCHI _____

27. KERAT _____

28. LAPAR _____

29. LARYNG _____

30. LIP _____

31. MAST _____

32. MEL _____

33. MYEL _____

34. MYO _____

35. NEPHYR _____

36. NEUR _____

37. ODONT _____

38. OPT _____

EXERCISES

Part C—cont'd

Match the following root words with the body parts that define their meaning.

39. OST _____

40. OT _____

41. PHLEB _____

42. POD _____

43. PROCT _____

44. RHIN _____

45. SPHYGM _____

46. STERN _____

47. THEL _____

48. TRACHEL _____

49. TRICH _____

■ LATIN ROOT WORDS A TO Z

In this section, we identify the more common root words that have their origins in Latin. The Latin roots are listed alphabetically followed by their meaning and examples. Exercises will follow.

AC, ACU (point)

acupuncture Technique that uses needles precisely placed into the tissue as a means of therapy to certain ailments

ACT, AG (to act)

agent Any substance that elicits a response

ADIP (fat)

adipocele Hernia with a hernial sac
adiposis Obesity, either local or widespread

AL (winged)

ala Any structure resembling a wing

ALB (white)

albinism Condition characterized as lacking pigment
albicant Tendency toward being white
albumin Protein found in animal tissue

ALVEOL (cavity)

alveolus Lung cell
labioalveolar Pertaining to the lip and jaw

AMBUL (to walk)

ambulance Vehicle used to transport patients
ambulatory Capable of walking

ANNUL (ring)

annulus Any ringlike structure
annulose Ringed

APIC (tip)

subapical Near the top
periapical Around the top

AQU (water)

subaqueous Below water
deaquation Elimination of water

ARC, ARCU (arched)

arciform Shaped as an arch

ARE (space)

areola Pigmented ring surrounding a central
area, as in a nipple

ARTICUL (joint)

interarticular Within the joint
biarticulate Double jointed

ATRI (room)

atrium Component of the heart

AUD (to hear)

anaudia Inability to speak associated with
hearing loss

AUR (ear)

aurist Specialty in the functioning of
the ears

AX (axis)

axiolabial Angle created by the axis formed from
the teeth and lips

BARB (beard)

barbate Having hair on the cheeks or jaw

BI, BIN (two)

binary fission Splitting of one cell into two equal
cells
biped Two footed
bisect To split in two

BILI (bile)

bilirubinemia Condition characterized by blood
with components of the bile

BUCC (cheek)

buccal Pertaining to the cheek
extrabuccal Outside the mouth

BULL (blister)

bulla Lymph-filled blister, usually within the
epidermis

CAL (to be warm)

calefacient Topical medication that causes
a sensation of warmth
calorie Unit of heat

CALC (calcium)

calcipenia Nutrition deficiency characterized by
a lack of calcium

CALCAR (spur)

calcarate Having a spurlike point

CALL (hardened skin)

callous Pertaining to a localized area of hard
skin

CAN (glowing)

incandescent Glowing hot

CAP, CAPT, CEPT (to receive)

susceptible State of being readily accepting of
pathogens or circumstance
capacious Containing a large quantity

CAPILL (hair)

capillovenous Meeting point of a venule and a capillary

capilliculture Hair-loss treatment

CAPS (box)

capsulitis Capsule inflammation

encapsulation Surrounding of a larger part by a capsule

CENT (one hundred)

centimeter One hundredth of a meter

CEREBR (brain)

cerebellum Part of the brain

cerebral Pertaining to the brain

CERN, CRET, CRE (to separate or to secrete)

secernment Glandular secretion

incretion Secreting internally

CERVIC (neck)

endocervicitis Inflammation of the inner cervical lining

cervicodynia Neck cramping

CESS (to yield)

recessive One set of traits that are less likely to appear in the phenotype than is the dominant trait

introcession Depression or dip in the surface

CID (to fall)

incidence Act or manner of falling

CING (to bind)

cingulum Waist

CIPIT (head)

bicipital In reference to biceps

occipital Pertaining to the back of the head

CIS (to cut)

circumcise Procedure to remove the male foreskin

CLAV (1) (club)

clavate Shaped so that one end is wider than the other

CLAV (2) (key)

clavicle Collarbone

CLIV (slope)

clivus Slope

declivous Sloping downward

CLUS, CLOS (to close)

preclusion Inability to perform movement

exclusion Rendering useless without removal

occlusion Being closed

COLL (neck)

collarbone Clavicle bone

CORD (heart)

postcordial Positioned at the rear of the heart or behind the heart

CORN (horny)

cornification Tissue deterioration to dead, horny tissue

subcorneous Beneath the horny layer

CORP, CORPUS (body)

corpse Dead body

corpuscle Small, round entity

CORT (the outermost layer)

cortex Outlying tissue of an organ

CRE, CRESC, CRET (to grow)

intercrescence To grow into one

concrement Merging of two things, usually found separate, as in toes

CUB (to lay down)

decubitus ulcer Reoccurring bedsore

CURR, CURS (to go)

succursal Secondary part to a greater whole

CUSPID (point)

cuspid Arriving at a rounded or pointed end
bicuspid Type of tooth with a double point

CUSS (to shake)

concussion Effect of being shaken
percussion Effect of firmly tapping the body to use
   the vibratory effects as a means of diagnosis

CUT (skin)

intracutaneous Within the skin
cutin Found in upper epidermis

DEC, DECIM (ten)

decimeter One tenth of a meter

DENT (tooth)

dentate Possessing teeth
dedentition Loss of teeth

DEXTR (to the right side)

dextroduction Eye movement to the right side
ambidextrous Ability to use both sides of the
   body with equal agility

DIGIT (toe and finger)

digital In reference to fingers and toes

DOL (to feel pain)

dolor Pain

DORM, DORMIT (to sleep)

dormitive Induces sleep

DORS (back)

dorsal Positioned in the rear

DUC, DUCT (to lead)

abduction Removal of a part from the whole
levoduction Eye movement to the left

DUR (hard)

epidural Situated on or near the dura mater
subdural Beneath the dura mater

EGO (I)

egomania Heightened sense of self-grandeur
egopathy Hostile consequence of imposing ones
   will on others

ERR (to wander or to deviate)

errant Tendency to stray from a usual pattern of
   movement
erratic Having an irregular course

FA (to speak)

infant One who does not speak, most often a
   child under the age of 2 years
infanticide Killing of an infant

FACI (surface)

bifacial Two distinct surfaces
interface Surface that acts as a boundary or a
   mediator between two other surfaces

FACT, FIC (to make)

artifact Any structure that has been made by
   artificial means
efficacious To have a desired end result

FASCI (band)

fascia Pertaining to a band of connective
   tissue
fascitis Inflammation of the fascia

FEBR (fever)

febrile Pertaining to or having a fever

FER (to carry or produce)

afferent To bring closer
lactiferous Capable of making milk
proliferate To grow with multiplicity

FERR (iron)

ferrihemoglobin Ferrous state of iron in the
hemoglobin

FIBR (fiber)

fibril Small component of the larger fiber
fibrin Protein that plays a role in blood clotting

FIBUL (clasp)

fibula Outer bone of the leg
parafibular Pertaining to the areas and functions
around the fibula

FIL (thread)

filament Tiny threadlike structures
filiform Shaped as filaments

FISS (to separate)

fissure Separation of internal tissues

FLAGELL (whip)

hemoflagellate Protozoan that resides in the
blood of its host

FLAV (yellow)

riboflavin Member of the vitamin B complex
flavedo Yellowing of the skin

FLEX (to bend)

reflex Fixed response to a given stimuli
dorsiflexion Movement of a joint toward the
posterior position of the body
circumflex To wind around

FLU, FLUX (to flow)

confluent Existing parallel of one another
reflux Back flow, opposite of the normal flow

FOLL (bag)

follicle Small sac with secretory functions
folliculitis Inflammation of a follicle

FRAC, FRAG (to break or to bend)

refract To cause a straight ray of light to bend
diffraction Splitting a ray of light into its various
components using a prism

FRUCT (fruit)

fructose Simple sugar found in fruit

FUN (cord)

funiculitis Inflammation of the funiculus
funic Pertaining to the umbilical cord

FUNG (fungus)

fungal Pertaining to fungi

FURC (fork)

trifurcate Having three branches
furcula Forked structure
bifurcate Having two branches

FUS (to pour)

infusion Injection of a fluid into the body
perfusion Movement of fluid through a certain
space
suffusion Spreading of fluid in a given space
effusion Escape of a fluid

FUSC (dark)

fuscin Dark pigment in the eye
obfuscation Incoherence or confusion

GEMIN (paired)

geminate To pair off
bigeminy Tendency to occur in pairs

GEN, GENU (knee)

genupectoral Positioned with the knees bent
upward toward the chest

GEST (to carry)

digestion Process of dissolving food for transport around the body

ingestion Process by which matter is taken into the body

GINGIV (gums)

gingival Pertaining to the gums

labiogingival Pertaining to lips and gums

GLAB, GLABR (smooth)

glabella Region on the forehead between the eyebrows

GRAV (heavy)

multigravida Pregnancy after prior pregnancies

primigravida First-time pregnancy

GREG (to flock)

gregarious Congregating in groups

GUST (to taste)

gustation Sense of taste

HAL, HALIT (to breath)

halitosis Condition characterized by chronic bad breath

inhale To breathe inward

HER, HES (to stick)

adhesion Holding together, as in sutures

adhesiotomy Surgical removal of an adhesion

incoherent Erratic or irregular

HIAT (to remain open)

hiatus Opening

I, IT (to go)

abient Tendency to move away from the source

ILE (ileum)

ileum Small intestine

INGUIN (groin)

inguinal Groin region

INSUL (island)

Insulin Hormone that is created by Langerhans cells within the pancreas

JACUL (to dart)

ejaculate Projection of the seminal fluid

JECT (to throw)

projectile Object that is cast away with speed and over distance

JUNCT, JUG (to join)

conjunction Meeting of two or more components in a single place

conjugation Joining of two unicellular organisms

conjunctivitis Inflammation of mucous membrane

LAB (to fall)

labile Moving about in an unstable manner

LABI (lip)

labium Liplike structure

LACRIM (tear)

lacrimal Pertaining to tears or tear ducts

nasolacrimal Pertaining to the tear-producing organs and the nose

LACT (milk)

lactation Production and secretion of milk from the mammary gland

lactase Enzyme that breaks down the sugar lactose

LAMELL (thin plate)

lamella Thin plate or layer

LAT (to carry)

ablation Amputation

LATER (side)

lateral Pertaining to the side
dorsolateral Pertaining to the side and the back
heterolateral Pertaining to the opposite side
bilateral Pertaining to both sides

LENT (lens)

lentiginose Polka dotted, speckled randomly

LEV (1) (to the right side)

levoduction Eye movement toward the right side

LEV (2) (lightweight)

levator Any agent that elevates

LIEN (spleen)

lienal Pertaining to the spleen

LIG (to bind)

ligature Cord for tying vessels
ligation Act of tying vessels with a ligature

LINE (line)

linear Sequential or in a logical manner
lineolate Marked with a reoccurring lined pattern, or stripped

LOB (lobe or ear)

lobotomy Cutting into the lobe

LUC (light)

translucid Opaque to transparent

LUM (light)

lumen Inner portion of a tubular structure
luminosity Ability to emit light

LUMB (loin)

lumbar Pertaining to the light

LUN (moon)

semilunar Shaped as a half moon
lunula White, half-moon shaped white portion of the nail near the root

MACUL (spot)

macula Spot of discoloration
emaculation Removal of freckles and spots, including skin tumors
maculopapular Pertaining to a spot and a papule

MAGN (large)

magnify To make appear larger
magnitude Pertaining to a particular size

MAL (cheek)

malar Pertaining to the cheek
maloplasty Corrective or plastic surgery on the cheeks or cheekbones

MAL, MALE (bad)

malocclusion Any formation of teeth other than what is normal
malpractice Poor treatment by either carelessness or mistake

MALLE (hammer)

malleus Hammer shaped
submalleate Resembling a hammer

MAMM (breast)

mammilla Nipple
mammillary Nipple shaped
mammillitis Inflammation of the nipple

MAN, MANU (hand)

bimanous Having two hands

MATR, MATERN (mother)

dura mater Fibrous tissue covering the spinal cord and brain

MEAT (to pass)

meatus An opening
meatitis Inflammation of the wall of the meatus

MEDI (middle)

mediodorsal Middle line on the back
mediad Toward the middle

MENT (1) (chin)

mental Pertaining to the chin

MENT (2) (mind)

mentation Active processes of the mind
amentia Below normal brain functioning
dementia Loss or decline in mental function

MIL, MILL (one thousand)

millimeter One thousandth of a meter

MOLL (soft)

molluscum Skin disease characterized by
    pus-filled nodules

MORT (death)

mortal Likely to cause death
postmortem After death

MOT (to move)

motile Having the ability to move

MUC (mucus)

mucocutaneous Pertaining to mucus membranes
    and the skin

MULT (many)

multiocular Vision with many eyes

MUR (wall)

mural Pertaining to a wall

NAR (nostril)

nariform Shaped as a nostril

NAS (nose)

nasal Pertaining to the nose
nasion The midpoint of the nasal region
postnasal Occurring behind the nose

NERV (nerve)

innervation Placement and distribution of nerves
abnerval Positioned away from a nerve

NEV (birthmark)

nevus Birthmark or mole

NIGR (black)

nigricant Blackish

NOCT (night)

noctiphobia Fear of the night or darkness

NOM (name)

binomial Having two names

NON, NOVEM (nine)

nonipara Woman who has had nine successful
    pregnancies

NUC (nut)

mononucleosis Condition characterized by an
    abnormally high quantity of leukocytes or
    monocytes in the bloodstream
nucivorous Having the ability of eating nuts

NUTRI, NUTRIT (to nourish)

nutrient Any of the required vitamins and
    minerals a body needs to function

OCT, OCTAV (eight)

octal Pertaining to the number eight

OCUL (pertaining to the eye)

oculomotor Pertaining to the functions that cause
    the eyeball to move
binocular Vision with the use of two eyes

ORB (circular)

orbiculate Circular in shape
exorbitism Protrusion of the eyeball from
    the socket

OS, OR (mouth)

osculation Joint between vessels
circumoral Around the mouth

OSS (bone)

ossicle Small bone
dermo-ossification Bone forming in the skin
ossify To turn to bone

OV (egg)

binovular Reference to two ovum, as with
    fraternal twinning

PALAT (palate)

palatitis Inflammation of the palate

PALP (to touch)

palpation Use of touch for diagnostic
    purposes
impalpable Unable to be detected by touch

PAR (to produce)

primapara First time giving birth
bipara Giving birth to two babies
    simultaneously

PAT (to open)

patent Pertaining to that which is open
patella Kneecap or the elbow

PATI (to suffer)

patient One who suffers from any disorder that
    requires specialized help

PECTOR (breast)

pectoral Pertaining to the chest or breast
mediopectoral Central area of the chest

PED (foot)

pedestrian Someone who travels by foot
pedicure Care and maintenance of the feet

PEL, PELL, PULS (to beat)

impulsion Drive to move forward
pulsion Pushing forward
pulse rate Rate at which the heart beats

PELL (skin)

pellicle Sheer, protective coating of skin

PET, PETIT (to seek)

impetigo Condition characterized by skin
    inflammation
inappetence Loss of desire

PIL (hair)

pilosebaceous Pertaining to the hair follicles and
    accompanying sebum secreting glands
pilose High hair density
pilocystic Hair and fat-encysted tumors
epilate To remove a hair from the root, causing
    damage to the follicle

PLANT (sole of the foot)

planta Sole of the foot

PLEX (to interweave)

plexus Network of nerves, blood vessels, or
    lymphatics
complex Grouping of related symptoms
plexure To weave or intertwine

PLIC, PLICIT (to fold)

plica Skin fold
complicate To fold

PLUR (more)

pluriparity Woman who has bore many
    children

POSIT (to put)

suppository Medication in the form of a soft
solid, administered by placement in an orifice

POT (sense of power)

potent Having strength
unipotent Embryonic cells that grow into only
one type of cell or tissue
potentiation Addition of more ingredients to
make the whole more potent

PRIM (first)

primigravida First-time pregnancy

PRON (face down)

prone Resting in a position such that the face is
down and the dorsal side is exposed
pronation State of being prone

PROXIM (near)

proximate Nearest or most likely cause

PRUR (to itch)

antipruritic Anything that relieves an itch
pruritus Itchiness caused by irritation of the
peripheral sensory nerve

PULMO, PULMON (lung)

gastropulmonary Pertaining to the lungs and
digestive tract
cardiopulmonary Pertaining to the heart and
lungs

PUNCT (point)

punctual Pertaining to a point

PUR (pus)

purulent Pus forming

QUADRU (four)

quadrivalent Association of four chromosomes
quadruped Four-legged animal

QUART (four)

quaternate Set of four

QUINQUE (five)

quinquepartite Having five parts

QUINT (five)

quintuplet Five children conceived and born at once

RADI (radius or ray)

radiotherapy Use of x-ray as a diagnostic tool or
other radioactive products in the treatment of
disease

REG, RECT (to make straight)

arrector Muscle that makes straight

REN (kidney)

adrenal Glands attached to the kidneys
reniform Kidney shaped

RET (net)

rete Network or web
retina Light-receptive layer in the eye

RIG (stiff)

rigid Stiff or hardened

RIM (crack)

birimose Having two cracks or slits

ROS (to eat away at)

corrosive Agent that destroys tissue
erosion Wearing away

ROT (round)

rotate Round in shape

RUB (red)

bilirubin Pigment of blood and bile
rubella German measles
erubescent Pink-red color or blushed

RUG (wrinkle)

erugatory Having the ability to remove wrinkles

RUPT (to break)

rupture Forceful tear

SALI, SILI, SULT (to jump)

insult Discontinuation of tissue

SANGUI (blood)

sanguimotor Pertaining to circulation of the blood through the body

SCRIB, SCRIPT (to write)

superscription Rx at the beginning of a prescription
subscription Part of a prescription that directs the formula, specifics
prescription Authorization for a patient to use a controlled substance for therapeutic purposes

SEB (grease)

sebum Secretion on the sebaceous glands
sebaceous Pertaining to sebum
seborrhea Condition characterized by overactive secretion of the sebaceous glands

SEC, SECT, SEG (to cut)

resection Process of cutting out, as in a growth
exsection Excision
bisect To split in two

SECOND, SECUND (second)

secundines Afterbirth
secundigravidas Woman's second pregnancy

SEMI (half)

semilunar Half moon

SEMIN (seed)

semination Dispersal of seeds
seminuria Urine mixed with semen

SEN (old)

senium Pertaining to old age

SEP, SEPT (1) (to separate)

septum Any partition or divider that separates a space or cavity

SEP, SEPT (2) (seven)

septimal Pertaining to seven
septuplets Seven children conceived and born at once

SESQUI (one and a half)

sesquioxide Any compound that has a 3:2 ratio of oxygen and another compound

SEXT (six)

sextant At an angle of at least 60 degrees

SICC (dry)

siccant Tendency toward being dry

SOL (sun)

solarization Use of artificial or natural sunlight for therapeutic purposes

SOLV, SOLUT (dissolve)

absolute Free from mixture
liposoluble Soluble in fat
solvent Substance capable of dissolving another substance

SOMN (sleep)

insomnia Inability to get to or maintain healthy sleep
hypersomnia Oversleeping

SON (sound)

asonia Inability to decipher tones
sonogram Instrument used to measure sound waves

SORB, SORPT (to draw inward)

absorption Ability to draw fluids inward

SPIC (cone)

spicula Small conical-shaped body

SPIN (thorn)

spinocellular Pertaining to prickle cells

SPIR (to breath)

respiration Process of taking in oxygen and
   circulating it around the body while
   removing carbon dioxide
suspiration Sighing

SQUAM (scale)

squamous Pertaining to flat, scaly epithelium cells

STA (to stand)

stable Agent that is unlikely to decompose

STRAT (layer)

stratum Layer of tissue
bistratose Cells organized in two layers
stratify To layer

STRI (striated)

stria Streak or a line

STRING, STRICT (to draw tight)

astringent Any agent that causes tissue to
   contract
restrict To constrict in such a manner that
   prevents fluid from making passage

STRU, STRUCT (to build)

ultrastructure Grouping of minute particles in an
   organized fashion

TACT (to touch)

tactile Pertaining to touch
atactilia Loss of the sense of touch

TEN, TENT (to hold)

incontinent Inability to control natural
   evacuation functions

TEND, TENS (to stretch)

tensor Muscle that makes a part tense

TERMIN (ending)

terminal Resulting in death
paraterminal Near an ending point

TERTI, TER, TERN (three)

tertiary Third stage, as in a disease

TRACT (to drag)

traction Use of pulling to regain muscle strength
extract To remove

TRI (third)

tricipital Having three heads

TRUS (to push)

extrusion To remove forcefully

TUBER (to swell)

tuber Subsurface root with a rounded outcropping
tubercle Having a nodule

TUM (to swell)

tumescent Swollen
tumentia Condition characterized by irregular
   swelling of the arms and legs

TUSS (cough)

tussive Pertaining to a cough

UN (one)

unipotent Embryonic cells that grow into only
   one type of cell or tissue

UNGU (nail)

unguiferate Having nails or claws

VAGIN (sheath)

vagina Canal leading to the uterus; the birthing canal

VAL (strength)

bivalent Applied to homologous pairs of chromosomes

VARI (varied)

varicella Chickenpox
varicelliform Resembling chickenpox

VARIC (swollen)

varicose Blood vessel that is twisted and bulbous, usually visible from the exterior of the body

VAS (vessel)

vasodilation Enlarging of blood vessels
cardiovascular Pertaining to the heart and blood vessels

VEN (vein)

rectivenous Having straight veins
intravenous Inside the veins

VENT (belly)

ventriculitis Inflammation of the ventricle linings within the brain
ventrose Swollen belly

VERI, VERT, VERS (to turn)

vericolor Multicolored
eversion Turning of the eyelid outwardly
transverse To position in the form of a cross
vertigo Dizziness

VESIC (blister)

vesication Formation of a blister

VISCER (entrails)

viscerotrophic Pertaining to the decomposition occurring in visceral conditions

VIT (life)

vitalism Theory suggesting that life is guided by a force greater than itself
vitamin Agent that improves life or quality of life

VITR (glass)

vitrescence State of being transparent and solid, as in glass
vitrification Act of making glass or making something glasslike

VULS (to tear)

avulsion Tear with force

EXERCISES

Part D

Identify the roots in each of the following words:

1. acupuncture _____

2. varicelliform _____

3. tumentia _____

4. adiposis _____

5. alveolus _____

6. albinism _____

Continued

EXERCISES

Part D—cont'd

Identify the roots in each of the following words:

7. annulus _____

8. periapical _____

9. deaquation _____

10. interarticular _____

11. astringent _____

12. areola _____

13. atrium _____

14. squamous _____

15. sonogram _____

16. anaudia _____

17. aurist _____

18. prescription _____

19. barbate _____

20. biped _____

21. extrabuccal _____

22. calefacient _____

23. radiotherapy _____

24. quinquepartite _____

25. purulent _____

26. erosion _____

27. calcipenia _____

28. seminuria _____

29. capacious _____

30. capilliculture _____

31. sebum _____

32. rigid _____

33. cerebral _____

34. rubella _____

35. incretion _____

36. multiocular _____

37. magnitude _____

38. linear _____

39. heterolateral _____

40. nasolacrimal _____

41. conjunctivitis _____

42. ejaculate _____

EXERCISES

Part D—cont'd

Identify the roots in each of the following words:

43. adhesiotomy _____

44. gingival _____

45. genupectoral _____

46. effusion _____

47. furcula _____

48. funiculitis _____

49. follicle _____

50. fissure _____

51. lactiferous _____

52. artifact _____

53. egopathy _____

54. levoduction _____

55. ambidextrous _____

56. dedentition _____

57. intracutaneous _____

58. percussion _____

59. cuspid _____

Part E

Determine a root that corresponds to the following numbers:

0.5: _____

1: _____

1.5: _____

2: _____

3: _____

4: _____

5: _____

6: _____

7: _____

8: _____

9: _____

10: _____

100: _____

1000: _____

EXERCISES

Part F

Write the correct Latin root next to the following body parts that define their meaning:

1. entrails _____

2. joint _____

3. ear _____

4. cheek _____

5. hardened _____

6. skin _____

7. hair _____

8. brain _____

9. neck _____

10. head _____

11. heart _____

12. tooth _____

13. fingers _____

14. knee _____

15. gums _____

16. groin _____

17. lip _____

18. spleen _____

19. breast _____

20. hand _____

21. chin _____

22. nostril _____

23. nose _____

24. nerve _____

25. birthmark _____

26. eye _____

27. mouth _____

28. bone _____

29. foot _____

30. lung _____

31. kidney _____

32. belly _____

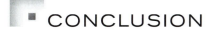

CONCLUSION

Having a firm grasp of root words is critical to mastery of medical terminology. Taking the time to memorize these words will help you accomplish as much. Cumulatively, the Greek and Latin roots form the crux of medical terminology. In the following chapters, we examine the prefixes and suffixes that complete the words. However, take the time to learn the roots first because you will be well served in following chapters.

CHAPTER REFERENCES

Ayers, D.M. (1972). *Bioscientific terminology: Words from Greek and Latin stems.* Phoenix: University of Arizona Press.

Chabner, D.E. (2003). *Medical terminology: A short course* (3rd ed.). Philadelphia: W. B. Saunders.

Medical terminology made easy. Available at *www.dictionary.com.*

Thomas, C.L., (Editor). (1997). *Taber's cyclopedic medical dictionary* (vol. 18). Philadelphia: F.A. Davis.

Prefixes

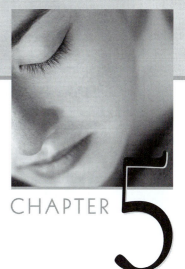

CHAPTER 5

LEARNING OBJECTIVES

After completing this chapter, you should be able to:

1. Identify the prefixes that are of Greek origin.
2. Identify the prefixes that are of Latin origin.
3. Define the meanings of prefixes.
4. Combine prefixes with root words already learned to make new words.

INTRODUCTION

By this point, we have explored the more common root words that you will encounter. These root words have their origins in the Greek and Latin languages. The same applies to prefixes.

Prefixes are words or word parts that are added to the root words to change their meaning. Some prefixes can modify the meaning; others are capable of completely changing the entire meaning. First, we will examine Greek prefixes, followed by Latin prefixes. Exercises will follow to further enhance your ability to comprehend.

GREEK PREFIXES A TO Z

In most instances, Greek prefixes are attached to words, as we have mentioned, which will modify or change their meanings. Originally, these prefixes stood alone as prepositions or adverbs. However, these words rarely stand alone anymore.[*] In many instances, these prefixes will end in a vowel. However, the vowel is dropped when the root word ends in an *h* or another vowel.

Prefixes, their meanings, and examples with which to begin working are listed here.

A, AN (not or without)

aphasia Loss of the ability to use words
anesthetic Any agent that blocks pain

AMPHI, AMPHO (both)

amphogenic Producing the same number of male and female children

ANA (up or again)

anastalsis Antiperistalsis
anastomosis Intercommunication of blood vessels related to blood pathways

ANTI (opposite)

antipruritic Anything that relieves an itch
antibiotic Relationship between two organisms in which one will kill the other

APO (away)

apophysis Projection of an organ
apoplexy Complex resulting from hemorrhaging from or onto the brain

CATA (down or against)

cataplexy Sudden muscular rigidity brought on by fear in some animals

DYS (bad or difficult)

dystrophy Inadequate or compromised nutrition
dysarthria Speech impairment

EC, EX (outward or outside)

excrement Discharge of useless substances from the body
ecmnesia Inability to recall short-term memory events

EN, EM, EL (inward)

embryo Unborn child during the first 3 months of gestation
environment Set of circumstances in which something exists

ENDO, ENTO (within)

endocrine Excreted internally

EPI (upon)

epidemic Disease that is rampant on a localized level
epidermis Outermost layer of skin

ES, EIS (into or inward)

esodic Afferent nerve that sends signals to the central nervous system

EU (normal)

eubiotics Science of hygiene and healthy lifestyles
euhydration Normal levels of water in the body

EXO, ECTO (external)

exocardial Occurring outside the heart
exocrine Excreted externally

---

[*]Ayers, D. (1972). *Bioscientific terminology: Words from Greek and Latin stems.* Phoenix, AZ: University of Arizona Press.

HYPER (more)

hypergia Increase in functional activity
hyperergy Sensitivity to allergens

HYPO (less)

hypogastropagus Conjoined twins joined at the stomach region
hypophrenia Having or relating to feeblemindedness

META (change or transfer)

metabiosis Relationship between two organisms in which one benefits (e.g., a black widow spider that kills her mate after seeding her eggs)

PARA (beside or associated with)

paraplegia Paralysis of the lower limbs
parafibular Pertaining to the areas and functions surrounding the fibula

PERI (around or nearby)

peripheral Related to, located in, or constituting an outer boundary
pericranium Outer surface of the cranial bones

PRO (before)

progeria Premature senility
prognosis Educated guess as to cause, course, and treatment of a given set of symptoms

PROS (toward or in addition to)

prosthodonthia Sect of dentistry that specializes in artificial tooth replacement

SYM (with or together)

asymmetrical Two sides that are not equal
symbiosis Union of two organisms for mutual benefit

EXERCISES

Part A

Match the following terms with the correct definition:

amphogenic	cataplexy	esodic	metabiosis
anastalsis	dysarthria	eubiotics	parafibular
anastomosis	dystrophy	euhydration	paraplegia
antibiotic	ecmnesia	excrement	pericranium
antipruritic	embryo	exocardial	peripheral
aphasia	endocrine	exocrine	progeria
apophysis	environment	hyperergy	
apoplexy	epidemic	hypergia	
asymmetrical	epidermis	hypogastropagus	

1. _____   Speech impairment

2. _____   Projection of an organ

3. _____   Science of hygiene and healthy lifestyles

Continued

EXERCISES

Part A—cont'd

Match the terms on the previous page with the correct definition:

4. _____   Inadequate or compromised nutrition

5. _____   Loss of the ability to use words

6. _____   Outside the heart

7. _____   Sudden muscular rigidity brought on by fear in some animals

8. _____   Anything that relieves an itch

9. _____   Increase in functional activity

10. _____   Inability to recall short-term memory events

11. _____   Related to, located in, or constituting an outer boundary

12. _____   Paralysis of the lower limbs

13. _____   Excreted internally

14. _____   Disease that is rampant on a localized level

15. _____   Discharge of useless substances from the body

16. _____   Afferent nerve that sends signals to the central nervous system

17. _____   Pertaining to the areas and functions surrounding the fibula

18. _____   Antiperistalsis

19. _____   Outermost layer of skin

20. _____   Two sides that are not equal

21. _____   Educated guess as to cause, course, and treatment of a given set of symptoms

EXERCISES

Part A—cont'd

Match the terms listed on page 79 with the correct definition:

22. _____   Relationship between two organisms in which one will kill the other

23. _____   Intercommunication of blood vessels related to blood pathways

24. _____   Conjoined twins joined at the stomach region

25. _____   Normal levels of water in the body

26. _____   Any agent that blocks pain

27. _____   Producing the same number of male and female children

28. _____   Complex resulting from hemorrhaging from or onto the brain

29. _____   Having or relating to feeblemindedness

30. _____   Set of circumstances in which something exists

31. _____   Outer surface of the cranial bones

32. _____   Relationship between two organisms in which one benefits

33. _____   Sensitivity to allergens

34. _____   Unborn child during the first 3 months of gestation

35. _____   Union of two organisms for mutual benefit

36. _____   Sect of dentistry that specializes in artificial tooth replacement

37. _____   Premature senility

38. _____   Excreted externally

EXERCISES

Part B

Match the correct meaning with the prefixes listed. Some answers will be used more than once.

around or nearby	both	less	up or again
away	change or transfer	more	upon
bad or difficult	down or against	normal	with or together
before	external	opposite	within
beside or associated	into or inward	outward or outside	
with	inward	toward or in addition to	

1. META _____

2. AMPHI _____

3. PROS _____

4. ENTO _____

5. PARA _____

6. EX _____

7. EU _____

8. EIS _____

9. PRO _____

10. A _____

11. AMPHO _____

12. HYPER _____

13. APO _____

14. EXO _____

15. ANA _____

16. EN _____

17. CATA _____

18. HYPO _____

19. ENDO _____

20. AN _____

21. SYM _____

22. EPI _____

23. ECTO _____

24. PERI _____

25. DYS _____

26. EC _____

27. EL _____

28. ANTI _____

29. ES _____

30. EM _____

EXERCISES

Part C

Decipher the meaning of the following words:

1. catatropia _____

   _____

2. endothelial _____

   _____

3. hypodactylia _____

   _____

4. peribronchial _____

   _____

5. hypodermic _____

   _____

6. symbrachydactyly _____

   _____

7. epiotic _____

   _____

8. dysgraphia _____

   _____

9. antigen _____

   _____

10. apoplexy _____

    _____

11. endocardial _____

    _____

12. aponeurology _____

    _____

13. exodontias _____

    _____

14. exogamy _____

    _____

15. anhydration _____

    _____

16. anamnesis _____

    _____

17. anaerobic _____

    _____

18. encephalic _____

    _____

Continued

EXERCISES

Part C—cont'd

Decipher the meaning of the following words:

19. encephalocele _____

_____

20. metaphrenia _____

_____

21. ectoderm _____

_____

22. metanephros _____

_____

23. antiparalytic _____

_____

24. amphicyte _____

_____

25. amphibious _____

_____

26. prosodemic _____

_____

27. entocele _____

_____

28. entopic _____

_____

29. paracrine _____

_____

30. parachromatism _____

_____

31. exanthema _____

_____

32. excerebration _____

_____

33. eucholia _____

_____

34. euglycemia _____

_____

35. episodic _____

_____

36. prophylactic _____

_____

EXERCISES

Part C—cont'd

Decipher the meaning of the following words:

37. procephalic _____

_____

38. acardia _____

_____

39. acephalus _____

_____

40. hyperpnea _____

_____

41. hyperphagia _____

_____

42. hyperphrenia _____

_____

LATIN PREFIXES A TO Z

Prefixes that are derived from Latin are used in much the same way Greek prefixes are used. They are added to other words to change or modify their meanings. Most Latin prefixes are Latin words from which the traditional Latin endings (*-a, -um,* and *-is*) have been removed.

For example, the Latin word *finis* means *end*. The *-is* ending is dropped, and we see the Latin base *fin* in English words such as *final*. Latin prefixes, similar to Greek prefixes, are often used interchangeably with Greek root words, meaning that many words can have a Latin prefix with a Greek root, or vice versa. Similarly, a base may be preceded by any number of prefixes that all collaborate with one another towards the goal of changing and modifying the root.

Prefixes, their meanings, and examples with which to begin working are listed here.

A, AB, ABS (from)

abnormal Deviating from that which would otherwise be expected under a given set of circumstances

abarthrosis Condition in which bones rub against one another

AD, AC, AG, AL (near, to or toward)

adrenal Near the kidneys

aggressive Course of progression that is more rapid or recurrent than would otherwise be expected

alleviate To relieve a symptom or symptoms

AMBI, AMBO (both)

ambidextrous Capable of using both right and left sides with equaled ease

ANTE (before)

antecedent Occurring beforehand

CIRCUM (around)

circumference Distance around
circumvent To take a path that intentionally avoids a sensitive area

COM, CON, CO (with)

complicate To fold
conjectiva Mucus membrane that lines the eyelid

CONTR (opposite)

contraceptive Any device intended to prevent pregnancy from occurring

DI, DIS, DIF (apart)

dissect To cut into two

E, EX, EF (out or complete)

excrement Discharge of useless substances from the body
external On the outside
calefacient Topical medication that causes a sensation of warmth

IM, IN (into)

insult Any event that causes the discontinuation of tissue
inappetence Loss of desire
impalpable Unable to be detected by touch

INFRA (below)

infrared Relating to the range of invisible radiation wavelengths from approximately 750 nanometers, slightly longer than red in the visible spectrum

INTER (between or among)

interarticular Within the joint
intercrescence Growing into one

INTRA, INTRO (within)

intraocular Within the eye cavity
intravenous Inside the veins
introcession Depression or dip in the surface

JUXA (on the side of or close to)

juxta-articular Positioned close to a joint

OB, OF, OP, OC (toward or completely)

obfuscation Incoherence or confusion
haematobic Living in the blood

PER (through or wrongly)

percussion Effect of firmly tapping the body to use the vibratory effects as a means of diagnosis
perfusion Movement of fluid through a certain space

POST (after or behind)

postcardial Positioned at the rear of the heart or behind the heart
postmortem After death
postnasal Occurring behind the nose

PRE (before)

prescription Authorization for a patient to use a controlled substance for therapeutic purposes
preclusion Inability to perform movement

PRO (forward or in front)

prognosis Educated guess as to cause, course, and treatment of a given set of symptoms
proliferate To grow with multiplicity
projectile Object that is cast away with speed and over distance

RE, RED (again)

resection Process of cutting out, as in a growth

respiration Act of taking in oxygen and circulating it around the body while removing carbon dioxide

RETRO (backward or back)

retrography Condition characterized by writing backwards

retronasal Positioned in the rear of the nasal cavity

SE (away)

secernment Glandular secretion

secrete To expel outward or discharge

SUB, SUC, SUF, SUP (under or somewhat)

subapical Near the top

subaqueous Below water

succursal Secondary part to a greater whole

suffusion The spreading of fluid in a given space

suppository Medication in the form of a soft solid administered by placement in an orifice

SUPER, SUPRA (above)

superscription Rx at the beginning of a prescription

TRANS, TRAN, TRA (across)

translucid Opaque to transparent

transverse To position in the form of a cross

ULTRA (beyond)

ultrasound Mechanism for diagnosis using sound waves

ultrastructure Grouping of minute particles in an organized fashion

EXERCISES

Part D

Match each of the following terms with the correct definitions on pages 88, 89, and 90:

ambidextrous	inappetence	postmortem	subapical
antecedent	infrared	postnasal	subaqueous
calefacient	insult	preclusion	succursal
circumference	interarticular	prescription	suffusion
circumvent	intercrescence	prognosis	superscription
complicate	intraocular	projectile	suppository
conjectiva	intravenous	proliferate	translucid
contraceptive	introcession	resection	transverse
dissect	juxta-articular	respiration	ultrasound
excrement	obfuscation	retrography	ultrastructure
external	percussion	retronasal	
haematobic	perfusion	secernment	
impalpable	postcardial	secrete	

Continued

| EXERCISES |

Part D—cont'd

Match each of the terms on the previous page with the correct definitions below and on pages 89 and 90:

1. _____   Opaque to transparent

2. _____   Relating to the range of invisible radiation wavelengths from about 750 nanometers, slightly longer than red in the visible spectrum

3. _____   Secondary part to a greater whole secondary part to a greater whole

4. _____   Authorization for a patient to use a controlled substance for therapeutic purposes

5. _____   Below water

6. _____   Incoherence or confusion

7. _____   Grouping of minute particles in an organized fashion

8. _____   Any device intended to prevent pregnancy from occurring

9. _____   Living in the blood

10. _____   Near the top

11. _____   To grow into one

12. _____   To cast away with speed and distance

13. _____   To cut into two

14. _____   Use of sound waves as a mechanism for diagnosis

15. _____   Depression or dip in the surface

16. _____   Positioned in the rear of the nasal cavity

EXERCISES

Part D—cont'd

Match each of the terms listed on page 87 with the correct definitions below and on page 90:

17. _____   To firmly tap the body to use the vibratory effects as a means of diagnosis

18. _____   Condition characterized by writing backwards

19. _____   To grow with multiplicity

20. _____   Within the joint

21. _____   Distance around

22. _____   Medication in the form of a soft solid, administered by placement in an orifice

23. _____   Positioned close to a joint

24. _____   Positioned at the rear of the heart or behind the heart

25. _____   Occurring beforehand

26. _____   Process of cutting out, as in a growth

27. _____   Discharge of useless substances from the body

28. _____   Rx at the beginning of a prescription

29. _____   To take a path that intentionally avoids a sensitive area

30. _____   Inability to perform movement

31. _____   Inside the veins

32. _____   Occurring behind the nose

33. _____   To position in the form of a cross

Continued

> **EXERCISES**

Part D—cont'd

Match each of the terms listed on page 87 with the correct definitions below:

34. _____ Loss of desire

35. _____ Movement of fluid through a certain space

36. _____ Within the eye cavity

37. _____ To fold

38. _____ Spreading of fluid in a given space

39. _____ On the outside

40. _____ Glandular secretion

41. _____ Act of taking in oxygen, and circulating it around the body while removing carbon dioxide

42. _____ Topical medication that causes a sensation of warmth

43. _____ To expel outward or discharge

44. _____ Capable of using both right and left sides with equaled ease

45. _____ Unable to be detected by touch

46. _____ Educated guess as to cause, course, and treatment of a given set of symptoms

47. _____ Mucous membrane that lines the eyelid

48. _____ After death

49. _____ Any event that causes the discontinuation of tissue

EXERCISES

Part E

Match the correct meaning with the prefixes listed.

above	backward or back	from	toward or completely
across	before	into	under or somewhat
after or behind	below	near to or toward	with
again	between or among	on the side of or close to	within
apart	beyond	opposite	
around	both	out or complete	
away	forward or in front	through or wrongly	

1. RETRO _____

2. AB _____

3. TRAN _____

4. SUF _____

5. ULTRA _____

6. COM _____

7. INTER _____

8. EF _____

9. JUXA _____

10. E _____

11. AL _____

12. PRO _____

13. INFRA _____

14. EX _____

15. SUC _____

16. SUPRA _____

17. ANTE _____

18. CIRCUM _____

19. CO _____

20. AG _____

21. TRANS _____

22. INTRO _____

23. OC _____

24. SUPER _____

25. A _____

26. CONTR _____

27. DI _____

28. SUB _____

Continued

> **EXERCISES**

Part E—cont'd

Match the correct meanings listed on the previous page with the following prefixes:

29. IM _____ 40. OP _____

30. IN _____ 41. DIF _____

31. DIS _____ 42. CON _____

32. PER _____ 43. POST _____

33. RED _____ 44. RE _____

34. INTRA _____ 45. SE _____

35. OB _____ 46. SUP _____

36. AC _____ 47. AD _____

37. AMBO _____ 48. AMBI _____

38. PRE _____ 49. TRA _____

39. ABS _____

> **EXERCISES**

Part F

Decipher the meaning of the following words:

1. retroflexion _____

   _____

2. ablactation _____

   _____

3. pediastole _____

   _____

4. opposition _____

   _____

EXERCISES

Part F—cont'd

Decipher the meaning of the following words:

5. postnecrotic _____

_____

6. percutaneous _____

_____

7. intrapartum _____

_____

8. transocular _____

_____

9. respiratory _____

_____

10. inscription _____

_____

11. constriction _____

_____

12. diffuse _____

_____

13. subpericardial _____

14. impotent _____

_____

15. ultrasonic _____

_____

16. abrachia _____

_____

17. interatrial _____

_____

18. introjection _____

_____

19. transmural _____

_____

20. trajectory _____

_____

21. antifebrile _____

_____

22. procephalic _____

_____

Continued

EXERCISES

Part F—cont'd

Decipher the meaning of the following words:

23. circumcision _____

_____

24. infraclavicular _____

_____

25. contralateral _____

_____

26. supergenual _____

_____

27. supraoccipital _____

_____

CONCLUSION

Prefixes can change or modify the meaning of a root. Therefore understanding their meanings is important, thus when dissecting a word, you can accurately decipher its meaning. Root words are most often of Greek or Latin origin. In their former states, these words used to be adverbs and prepositions. Today, in English and medical terminology, the portions of words serve the same purpose, but they are added to the word itself. Knowing the meanings of these prefixes is critical to the comprehension of medical terminology.

CHAPTER REFERENCE

Ayers, D. (1972). *Bioscientific terminology: Words from Greek and Latin stems.* Phoenix, AZ: University of Arizona Press.

Suffixes

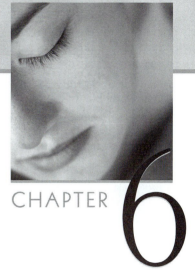

LEARNING OBJECTIVES

After completing this chapter, you should be able to:

1. Identify the suffixes that are of Greek origin.
2. Identify the suffixes that are of Latin origin.
3. Define the meanings of suffixes.
4. Combine suffixes with root words already learned to make new words.

INTRODUCTION

J ust as prefixes occur in front of words, suffixes occur at the end of words. Similar to prefixes, suffixes also modify a words meaning. Unlike prefixes, suffixes also help determine whether the word is an adjective, verb, or a noun. For example, the root word *gen* or *gene* means *to produce*. Gene, a form of the root aforementioned, is a noun. However, the word genetic is an adjective. Knowing the meaning of a suffix is just as important as is knowing the root word and the prefix in discerning the meaning of a medical term.

When dissecting a term for interpretation, you should start at the suffix, if the word has one. If a suffix is present, the process of unlocking its meaning begins with the clues given by the suffix. As mentioned, the most important clue the suffix provides is the part of speech of the word in question.

First, we will examine Greek suffixes, followed by Latin suffixes. Exercises will follow to further enhance your ability to comprehend.

GREEK SUFFIXES A TO Z

AL (pertaining to or similar to)

topical Applied externally
chondrosternal Pertaining to the chest and surrounding areas
metacarpal Part of the hand between the wrist and the digits

AN (pertaining to)

amphigean Native to all parts of the world

ARY (placement for)

malary Placed in the region of the cheeks
mammary Located on the breast
ovary Located near the ovum

ATE (to make)

carbohydrate Nutrient involved in the metabolism of food into energy
biarticulate Double jointed

ECTOMY (removal of)

hysterectomy Removal of the uterus
mastectomy Removal of the breast

EMIA (condition affecting the blood)

hypophrenia Having or relating to feeblemindedness
bilirubinemia Condition characterized by blood with components of the bile

GENOUS, GENIC (producing)

cryptogenic Of unknown etymology
pathogenic Capable of producing disease

IA, Y (state of)

arthralgia Joint pain
heteradenia Abnormal formation of a gland

IASIS (diseased condition)

psoriasis Chronic skin disease

IC, TIC (pertaining to or similar to)

synthetic Man made
polycystic Having many cysts

ICIAN (specializing in)

physician Person who treats illness or disease
optician Person who treats diseases of the eye

ICS, TICS (the study of)

genetics Study of genes and heredity
presbyatrics Field of study dealing with the diseases associated with old age
pediatrics Pertaining to the study of childhood disease

ID, IDA, IDEA (related to)

multigravida Pregnancy after prior pregnancies
primigravida First-time pregnancy
translucid Opaque to transparent

IN, INE (chemical derivative of)

saline Salt water
hyaline Clear material found in bodily colloids and jellies
secundines Afterbirth

ISK, ISCUS (little)

laryngicus Condition characterized by having restricted larynges

ISM, ISMUS (condition of)

meniscus Shaped as a crescent
phlebismus Condition of the blood

IST, AST (one who)

psychiatrist Person who specializes in diseases of the mind
phlebotomist Person who specializes in blood-based procedures

ITIS (inflammation of)

acromastitis Inflammation of the nipple
bronchitis Inflammation of bronchial tubes
chorditis Inflammation of the spermatic cord

IUM (1) (part of, lining for, or in the area of)

endothelium Lining of blood vessels
epithelium Tissue that forms the epidermis
perinephrium Connective tissue of the kidney

IUM (2), ION (little)

bacterium Plural for bacteria; single-celled
   organisms
stomion Fissure of closed lips

IZE (to make or to treat)

cauterize To treat using heat as a mechanism

LOGY (the study of)

terminology Study of words and word origin
syndesmology Study of ligaments
psychobiology Psychology in relation to biology

LYSIS (dissolution by)

pyretolysis Fever reduction
phleboclysis Process of flushing a vein using
   saline
glycolysis Conversion of carbohydrates into lactic
   or pyruvic acid

MA, ME, M (the consequences or results of)

edema Swelling caused by fluid accumulation
   within tissue
exanthema Eruption outside the body, or on the
   skin

MANIA (madness or insanity about)

megalomania Having a high opinion of oneself

METER (measure)

centimeter One hundredth of a meter
decimeter One tenth of a meter
goniometer Instrument used to measure angles

METRY (study of measure)

geometry Study of angles and shapes

NOMY (study of)

astronomy Study of the stars, planets, and other
   celestial entities

ODE, OID (in the shape of)

iridochoroiditis Inflammation of the choroids and
   the iris
hyaloid Clear or glasslike

OMA (tumor resulting from or contained within)

condyloma Tumor resembling a wart
sarcoma Malignant tumor on connective
   tissues

OSIS (characterized as being diseased)

anastomosis Intercommunication of blood vessels
   related to blood pathways
adiposis Obesity, either local or widespread
halitosis Condition characterized by chronic bad
   breath

OUS (full of or pertaining to)

phyllopodous Having leaflike feet
digonoporous Male and female genital apertures
stenostomatous Narrow mouth

PATHY (disease of)

aeropathy Any disorder caused by a change in
   pressure
adenopathy Any disease of the glands
egopathy Hostile consequence of imposing a
   person's will on others

PHILIC, PHILOUS (loving)

anthropophilic Preferring humans over other
   animals

PHOBIA (fear of)

basophobia Fear of walking
gerontophobia Extreme fear of aging
dysmorphophobia Fear of deformation

PLASTY (formation of)

hetero-osteoplasty Grafting of a bone using the bone of another animal

rhinoplasty Plastic surgery done to reshape the tissue in or around the nose

RRHEA (abnormal flow)

diarrhea Abnormal flow of excrement

seborrhea Condition characterized by overactive secretion of the sebaceous glands

SCOPE, SCOPY (to see)

microscope Device used to see items too small to be seen by the unaided eye

laparoscopy Device used to view inside the abdomen

SIS, SIA, SY, SE (process by which)

asterognosis Inability to recognize objects by touch

phleboclysis To flush a vein using saline

hypodermoclysis Introduction of large quantities of fluid into subcutaneous tissues

STOMY (surgical opening of)

coloproctostomy Surgical creation of a new passage from the colon to the rectum

T, TE (one who or that which)

gamete Egg after fertilization

antidote Any agent that is used as a remedy for a given set of symptoms

TER (means for placement of)

ureter Passageway from the kidneys to the bladder

THERAPY (remedy for or by)

radiotherapy Treatment involving the use of light rays and x-rays

pyrotherapy Treatment that produces an adjunct remedy using heat

TOMY (surgery on or by)

hysterotomy Cesarean section

laparotomy Any surgery involving an incision into the abdomen

neurotomy Division of a nerve

URIA (condition affecting urine)

ischuria Retention of urine

polyuria Passage of excessive amounts of urine

albuminuria Presence of albumin in the urine

US (member of or person who)

alveolus Lung cell

annulus Any ringlike structure

EXERCISES

Part A

Match the terms below and on page 99 with the definitions provided.

acromastitis	anastomosis	bacterium	centimeter
adenopathy	annulus	basophobia	chondrosternal
adiposis	anthropophilic	biarticulate	chorditis
aeropathy	antidote	bilirubinemia	coloproctostomy
albuminuria	arthralgia	bronchitis	condyloma
alveolus	asterognosis	carbohydrate	cryptogenic
amphigean	astronomy	cauterize	decimeter

EXERCISES

Part A—cont'd

Match the terms below and on the previous page with the definitions provided.

diarrhea
digonoporous
dysmorphophobia
edema
egopathy
endothelium
epithelium
exanthema
gamete
genetics
geometry
gerontophobia
glycolysis
goniometer
heteradenia

hetero-osteoplasty
hyaline
hyaloid
hypodermoclysis
hypophrenia
hysterectomy
hysterotomy
iridochoroiditis
ischuria
laparotomy
laryngicus
malary
mammary
mastectomy
megalomania

meniscus
metacarpal
multigravida
optician
ovary
pathogenic
pediatrics
perinephrium
phlebismus
phlebotomist
physician
polycystic
presbyatrics
primigravida
psoriasis

psychiatrist
pyretolysis
saline
sarcoma
seborrhea
secundines
stomion
syndesmology
synthetic
terminology
topical
translucid
ureter

1. _____ Person who treats diseases of the eye

2. _____ Person who treats illness or disease

3. _____ Having many cysts

4. _____ Man made

5. _____ Chronic skin disease

6. _____ Abnormal formation of a gland

7. _____ Joint pain

8. _____ Capable of producing disease

9. _____ Of unknown etymology

10. _____ Condition characterized by blood with components of the bile

Continued

EXERCISES

Part A—cont'd

Match the terms on pages 98 and 99 with the definitions provided.

11. _____   Having or relating to feeblemindedness

12. _____   Removal of the breast

13. _____   Double jointed

14. _____   Nutrient involved in the metabolism of food into energy

15. _____   Located near the ovum

16. _____   Located on the breast

17. _____   Placed in the region of the cheeks

18. _____   Native to all parts of the world

19. _____   Part of the hand between the wrist and the digits

20. _____   Pertaining to the chest and surrounding areas

21. _____   Applied externally

22. _____   The study of genes and heredity

23. _____   Field of study dealing with the diseases associated with old age

24. _____   Pertaining to the study of childhood disease

25. _____   Pregnancy after prior pregnancies

26. _____   First-time pregnancy

27. _____   Opaque to transparent

28. _____   Salt water

EXERCISES

Part A—cont'd

Match the terms on pages 98 and 99 with the definitions provided.

29. _____   Clear material found in bodily colloids and jellies

30. _____   Obesity, either local or widespread

31. _____   Afterbirth

32. _____   Shaped as a crescent

33. _____   Inflammation of bronchial tubes

34. _____   Condition of the blood

35. _____   Person who specializes in blood-based procedures

36. _____   Condition characterized by chronic bad breath

37. _____   Inflammation of the nipple

38. _____   Tissue that forms the epidermis

39. _____   Lining of blood vessels

40. _____   Connective tissue of the kidney

41. _____   Plural for bacteria; single-celled organisms

42. _____   Inflammation of the spermatic cord

43. _____   The fissure of closed lips

44. _____   One tenth of a meter

45. _____   The study of angles and shapes

46. _____   Instrument used to measure angles

Continued

EXERCISES

Part A—cont'd

Match the terms on pages 98 and 99 with the definitions provided.

47. _____   To treat using heat as a mechanism

48. _____   Intercommunication of blood vessels related to blood pathways

49. _____   Malignant tumor on connective tissues

50. _____   The study of the stars, planets, and other celestial entities

51. _____   Tumor resembling a wart

52. _____   Clear or glasslike

53. _____   Inflammation of the choroids and the iris

54. _____   Person who specializes in diseases of the mind

55. _____   The study of words and word origin

56. _____   The study of ligaments

57. _____   Fever reduction

58. _____   To flush a vein using saline

59. _____   Swelling caused by fluid accumulation within tissue

60. _____   An eruption outside the body, or on the skin

61. _____   Substance abuse

62. _____   One hundredth of a meter

63. _____   Having a high opinion of oneself

EXERCISES

Part B

Match the following definitions with the prefixes. Some meanings will be used more than once.

abnormal flow
characterized as being
   diseased
chemical derivative of
condition affecting the
   blood
condition affecting
   urine
condition of
consequences or
   results of
disease of

dissolution by
fear of
formation
full of or pertaining to
in the shape of
inflammation of
little
loving
madness or insanity
   about
means for placement
   of

measure
member of or person
   who
one who
one who specializes in
one who or that which
part of, lining for, or
   in the area of
pertaining to or
   similar to
placement for
process by which

related to
remedy for or by
removal of
state of
study of
study of measure
surgery on or by
surgical opening of
to make
to make or to treat
tumor resulting from
   or contained within

1. PHOBIA   _____

2. STOMY   _____

3. THERAPY _____

4. IZE   _____

5. PHILOUS _____

6. ODE   _____

7. LOGY   _____

8. NOMY   _____

9. METER   _____

10. TER   _____

11. US   _____

12. LYSIS   _____

13. M   _____

14. PLASTY   _____

15. SE   _____

16. PHILIC   _____

17. OID   _____

18. SIS   _____

19. MANIA   _____

20. ARY   _____

21. TE   _____

22. MA   _____

23. ISK   _____

24. PATHY   _____

Continued

EXERCISES

Part B—cont'd

Match the definitions on previous page with the prefixes. Some meanings will be used more than once.

25. INE   _____

26. SY   _____

27. IN   _____

28. OUS   _____

29. ISCUS   _____

30. T   _____

31. URIA   _____

32. TOMY   _____

33. IC   _____

34. ISMUS   _____

35. SIA   _____

36. THERAPY   _____

37. TIC   _____

38. AST   _____

39. IST   _____

40. ID   _____

41. OMA   _____

42. ISM   _____

43. METRY   _____

44. ITIS   _____

45. IDA   _____

46. OSIS   _____

47. IUM   _____

48. AL   _____

49. ICS   _____

50. RRHEA   _____

51. ION   _____

52. ATE   _____

53. ECTOMY   _____

54. EMIA   _____

55. Y   _____

56. IA   _____

57. ICIAN   _____

58. AN   _____

59. TICS   _____

60. IDEA   _____

LATIN SUFFIXES A TO Z

Suffixes that are derived from the Latin language operate in much the same way that suffixes that are derived from the Greek language. They modify or change the meaning, in addition to deciphering which part of speech they will become. As such, suffixes are attached to the end of roots to accomplish as much. Exercises will follow to further enhance your ability to comprehend.

ABLE, IBLE (able to)

impalpable Unable to detect by touch
stable Agent that is unlikely to decompose
susceptible State of being readily accepting of pathogens or circumstance

ACEOUS (belonging to or resembling)

pilosebaceous Pertaining to the hair follicles and accompanying sebum-secreting glands
sebaceous Pertaining to sebum

ACIOUS (inclination toward)

capacious Containing a large quantity
efficacious Having a desired end result

AL, IAL, EAL, UAL (pertaining to)

adrenal Glands attached to the kidneys
punctual Pertaining to a point
septimal Pertaining to seven

AN, ANE (pertaining to)

subcutaneous Beneath the skin
intracutaneous Within the skin

ANCE, ANCY (state of being, quality of being)

substance Any agent that has an effect
appearance Way something seems from a visual perspective
pregnancy Period of gestation
ambulance Vehicle used to transport patients

ANT, IANT (to be)

malignant Capable of causing death or damage

AR (pertaining to)

parafibular Pertaining to the areas and functions related to the fibula
unicellular Composed of only one cell

ARY (pertaining to)

mammary Pertaining to the breast
gastropulmonary Pertaining to the lungs and digestive tract
cardiopulmonary Pertaining to the heart and lungs

ATE, ITE (characterized by having)

quaternate Set of four
rotate To move in a circular fashion

BUL, BULA, BLE, BULUM (resulting from, act of, or placement of)

dysbulia Inability to harness willpower

CRUM (means of or resulting from)

fulcrum Point at which a lever moves
involvcrum Sheath or a protective covering

CULE, CLE (small)

tubercle Nodule
ventricle Small cavity
testicle Male gonad

CULUM (resulting from or act of)

tentaculum Tactile hair

EL, ELLE (small)

vessel Small canal, tube, or duct meant to transport fluids
organelle Part of a cell meant to perform a specific function

ELLUS, ELLA, ELLUM (small)

cerebellum Part of the brain

ENCE, ENCY (state of being, quality of being)

inappetence Loss of desire
incidence Act or manner of falling
intercrescence To grow into one

ENT, IENT (to be)

afferent Bearing or conducting inward
confluent Existing parallel of one another
incoherent Erratic or irregular

ESCE (to begin or to be somewhat)

incandescence Glowing hot

ETTE, ET (small)

lancet Device used to puncture the skin

FORM (having the shape of)

arciform Shaped as an arch
filiform Shaped as filaments
nariform Shaped as a nostril

FY, FIC (to make or to cause)

ossify To turn into bone or bonelike material
vitrification Making glass or making like glass

IA (state of being or act of doing)

mitochondria Powerhouse within cells
amnesia Long-term memory loss

IC, TIC (pertaining to)

optic Pertaining to the eye
diotic Affecting both ears
exophthalmic Abnormal protrusion of the eyeball from its socket

ID (inclination toward)

rigid Stiff or hardened
translucid Opaque to transparent

IGATE, EGATE (to drive)

irrigate To flush out with fluid

IL (small)

fibril Small fibers

ILE (1), IL (pertaining to)

febrile Pertaining to or having a fever
tactile Pertaining to touch

ILE (2) (able to)

projectile Object that is cast away with speed and over distance
motile Moving
labile Moving about in an unstable manner

ILLUS, ILLA, ILLUM (small)

mammilla Nipple

IN (pertaining to)

luminosity Ability to emit light
vitamin Agent that improves life or quality of life

ION (act of or resulting from)

absorption Ability to draw fluids inward
erosion Process of wearing away
resection Process of cutting out, as in a growth

ITIOUS (characterized by)

excrementitious Pertaining to or similar to excrement

ITUDE (state of or able to)

aptitude Natural inclination toward something
magnitude Pertaining to a particular size

ITY, ETY, TY (state of being or quality of)

rigidity Tending to be rigid
pluriparity Woman who has bore many children

IVE (inclination toward)

tussive Pertaining to a cough

connective Having the ability to connect one material to another

refractive Causing a straight ray of light to bend

(U)LENT, (O)LENT (full of or predisposed to)

purulent Pus forming

quadrivalent Association of four chromosomes

MEN, MIN (resulting from or act of)

specimen Sample or an example

regimen Systematic or regular process

MENT, MENTUM (resulting from or act of)

excrement Needless materials that are removed from the body

momentum Characteristic of having and maintaining a certain pace

OR (1) (one who or that which)

incisor Tooth adapted for cutting

motor Ability to move

OR (2) (state of being or resulting from)

error Mistake

tumor Abnormal tissue growth

ORY (1) (inclination toward)

erugatory Having the ability to remove wrinkles

ambulatory Capable of walking

ORY (2) (placement for)

suppository Medication in the form of a soft solid, administered by placement in an orifice

OSE (full of)

bistratose Organized in two layers

varicose vein Blood vessel that is twisted and bulbous, visible usually from the exterior of the body

ventrose Swollen

OUS, IOUS, EOUS (1) (full of)

fibrous Many fibers

callous Pertaining to a localized area of hard skin

melanotrichous Dark haired

OUS (2) (inclination toward)

nervous Having a tendency toward excitement or panic

TRUM (means of or resulting from)

spectrum Range of values of a quantity or set of related quantities

ULE, OLE, LE (small)

nodule Small mass of tissue

venule Small vein

systole Contraction of the heart

ULOUS (inclination toward)

tremulous Tendency to tremble

ULUS, ULA, ULUM, OLA (small)

funiculus Small cord

specula Small, pointed structure

areola Pigmented ring surrounding a central area, as in a nipple

UNCLE (small)

carbuncle Small subcutaneous skin infection

furuncle Boil

UNCULUS (small)

pedunculus Stalk or stalklike structure

URE (act of or resulting from)

rupture Forceful tear

temperature Fever

US (act of or resulting from)

clivus Slope
tonus Normal muscle state characterized by
   partial contraction

Y (state of being or act of doing)

horny Mass of hardened tissue
bigeminy Tendency to occur in pairs

EXERCISES

Part C

Match the following terms with the correct definitions provided on pages 109 through 115:

absorption	exophthalmic	mitochondria	septimal
adrenal	febrile	momentum	specimen
afferent	fibril	motile	spectrum
ambulance	fibrous	motor	specula
ambulatory	filiform	nariform	stable
amnesia	fulcrum	nervous	subcutaneous
appearance	funiculus	nodule	substance
aptitude	furuncle	optic	suppository
arciform	gastropulmonary	organelle	susceptible
areola	horny	ossify	systole
bigeminy	impalpable	parafibular	tactile
bistratose	inappetence	pedunculus	temperature
callous	incandescence	pilosebaceous	tentaculum
capacious	incidence	pluriparity	testicle
carbuncle	incisor	pregnancy	tonus
cardiopulmonary	incoherent	projectile	translucid
cerebellum	intercrescence	punctual	tremulous
clivus	intracutaneous	purulent	tubercle
confluent	involvcrum	quadrivalent	tumor
connective	irrigate	quaternate	tussive
diotic	labile	refractive	unicellular
dysbulia	lancet	regimen	varicose
efficacious	luminosity	resection	ventricle
erosion	magnitude	rigid	ventrose
error	malignant	rigidity	venule
erugatory	mammary	rotate	vessel
excrement	mammilla	rupture	vitamin
excrementitious	melanotrichous	sebaceous	vitrification

EXERCISES

Part C—cont'd

Match the terms on the previous page with the correct definitions below and on pages 110 through 115:

1. _____   Round in shape

2. _____   Set of four

3. _____   Mistake

4. _____   Pertaining to the heart and lungs

5. _____   Pertaining to the lungs and digestive tract

6. _____   Pertaining to the breast

7. _____   Tendency to occur in pairs

8. _____   Composed of only one cell

9. _____   Abnormal tissue growth

10. _____   Pertaining to the areas and functions related to the fibula

11. _____   Mass of hardened tissue

12. _____   Capable of causing death or damage

13. _____   Vehicle used to transport patients

14. _____   Period of gestation

15. _____   Way something seems from a visual perspective

16. _____   Normal muscle state characterized by partial contraction

17. _____   Any agent that has an effect

Continued

Part C—cont'd

Match the terms on page 108 with the correct definitions below and on pages 111 through 115:

18. _____   Ability to move

19. _____   Loss of desire

20. _____   Small canal, tube, or duct meant to transport fluids

21. _____   Slope

22. _____   Tooth adapted for cutting

23. _____   Within the skin

24. _____   Fever

25. _____   Beneath the skin

26. _____   Pertaining to seven

27. _____   Pertaining to a localized area of hard skin

28. _____   Forceful tear

29. _____   Pertaining to a point

30. _____   Glands attached to the kidneys

31. _____   Inability to harness willpower

32. _____   Having desired end result

33. _____   Having a tendency toward excitement or panic

34. _____   Having and maintaining a certain pace

35. _____   Many fibers

EXERCISES

Part C—cont'd

Match the terms on page 108 with the correct definitions below and on pages 112 through 115:

36. _____   Pertaining to a particular size

37. _____   Point at which a lever moves

38. _____   Pertaining to or similar to excrement

39. _____   Association of four chromosomes

40. _____   Containing a large quantity

41. _____   Part of the brain

42. _____   Process of removing needless materials from the body

43. _____   Boil

44. _____   Pertaining to sebum

45. _____   Unable to detect by touch

46. _____   Pertaining to the hair follicles and accompanying sebum secreting glands

47. _____   Stalk or stalklike structure

48. _____   Tactile hair

49. _____   Natural inclination toward something

50. _____   Both ears

51. _____   State of being readily accepting of pathogens or circumstance

52. _____   Nipple

Continued

EXERCISES

Part C—cont'd

Match the terms on page 108 with the correct definitions below and on pages 113 through 115:

53. _____   Small subcutaneous skin infection

54. _____   Part of a cell meant to perform a specific function

55. _____   Systematic or regular process

56. _____   Abnormal protrusion of the eyeball from its socket

57. _____   Pigmented ring surrounding a central area, as in a nipple

58. _____   Sample or an example

59. _____   Male gonad

60. _____   Pus forming

61. _____   Small, pointed structure

62. _____   Agent that is unlikely to decompose

63. _____   Dark haired

64. _____   Making glass or making like glass

65. _____   Small cavity

66. _____   Causing a straight ray of light to bend

67. _____   Opaque to transparent

68. _____   Agent that improves life or quality of life

69. _____   Woman who has bore many children

70. _____   Having the ability to connect one material to another

EXERCISES

Part C—cont'd

Match the terms on page 108 with the correct definitions below and on pages 114 and 115:

71. _____ Moving

72. _____ Swollen

73. _____ To turn into bone or bonelike

74. _____ Ability to emit light

75. _____ Pertaining to a cough

76. _____ Shaped as a nostril

77. _____ Erratic or irregular

78. _____ Small cord

79. _____ Sheath or a protective covering

80. _____ Ability to draw fluids inward

81. _____ Blood vessel that is twisted and bulbous, visible
usually from the exterior of the body

82. _____ Moving about in an unstable manner

83. _____ Stiff or hardened

84. _____ Organized in two layers

85. _____ Nodule

86. _____ Shaped as filaments

87. _____ Process of cutting out, as in a growth

88. _____ Device used to puncture the skin

Continued

EXERCISES

Part C—cont'd

Match the terms on page 108 with the correct definitions below and on page 115:

89. _____   Pertaining to touch

90. _____   Wearing away

91. _____   Object that is cast away with speed and over distance

92. _____   Medication in the form of a soft solid, administered by placement in an orifice

93. _____   Pertaining to the eye

94. _____   Tendency to tremble

95. _____   Powerhouse within cells

96. _____   Contraction of the heart

97. _____   Act or manner of falling

98. _____   Existing parallel of one another

99. _____   Small fibers

100. _____   Tending to be rigid

101. _____   Small vein

102. _____   Shaped as an arch

103. _____   Capable of walking

104. _____   Pertaining to or having a fever

105. _____   Long-term memory loss

106. _____   Small mass of tissue

EXERCISES

Part C—cont'd

Match the terms on page 108 with the correct definitions below:

107. _____   Having the ability to remove wrinkles

108. _____   Range of values of a quantity or set of related
quantities

109. _____   Glowing hot

110. _____   To flush out with fluid

111. _____   To bring closer

Part D

Match the following definitions with the prefixes. Some meanings will be used more than once and some
prefixes will have more than one meaning.

able to	means of or resulting	small	state of or able to
act of or resulting	from	state of being or act of	to be
from	one who or that which	doing	to begin or to be
characterized by	pertaining to	state of being or	somewhat
full of or predisposed to	placement for	quality of	to drive
having the shape of	resulting from, act of,	state of being or	to make or to cause
inclination toward	or placement of	resulting from	

1. ABLE   _____   7. ARY   _____

2. AL   _____   8. ATE   _____

3. ANCE   _____   9. BLE   _____

4. ANE   _____   10. BUL   _____

5. ANT   _____   11. CLE   _____

6. AR   _____   12. CRUM   _____

Continued

EXERCISES

Part D—cont'd

Match the definitions on previous page with the prefixes that follow. Some meanings will be used more than once and some prefixes will have more than one meaning.

13. CULUM _____

14. EAL _____

15. EGATE _____

16. EL _____

17. ELLE _____

18. ELLUM _____

19. ELLUS _____

20. ENCE _____

21. ENT _____

22. EOUS _____

23. ESCE _____

24. ETTE _____

25. ETY _____

26. FIC _____

27. FORM _____

28. FY _____

29. IA _____

30. IAL _____

31. IANT _____

32. IBLE _____

33. IC _____

34. ID _____

35. IENT _____

36. IGATE _____

37. IL _____

38. ILE _____

39. ILLA _____

40. ILLUM _____

41. IN _____

42. ION _____

43. IOUS _____

44. ITE _____

45. ITIOUS _____

46. ITUDE _____

47. ITY _____

48. IVE _____

EXERCISES

Part D—cont'd

Match the definitions on page 115 with the prefixes that follow. Some meanings will be used more than once and some prefixes will have more than one meaning.

49. LE   _____

50. LENT   _____

51. MEN   _____

52. MENT   _____

53. MIN   _____

54. OLA   _____

55. OLE   _____

56. OR   _____

57. ORY   _____

58. OSE   _____

59. OUS   _____

60. TIC   _____

61. TRUM   _____

62. TY   _____

63. UAL   _____

64. ULE   _____

65. ULOUS   _____

66. ULUM   _____

67. ULUS   _____

68. UNCLE   _____

69. UNCULUS   _____

70. UOUS   _____

71. URE   _____

72. US   _____

73. Y   _____

CONCLUSION

Suffixes play a pivotal role in the interpretation of medical terminology. They determine the part of speech of the word and offer more clues by way of the individual meaning of the suffix. A word can have several derivatives that all may seem similar on the onset. However, knowing the meaning of the suffix is the first step to unlocking the meaning of the word.

By this point, we have examined root words, prefixes, and suffixes. These different word parts can often be mixed and matched to make up many more words. In the following chapter, we will offer the now more-advanced student of medical terminology some adjunct information that will also be beneficial.

CHAPTER REFERENCES

Ayers, D.M. (1972). *Bioscientific terminology: Words from Greek and Latin stems*. Phoenix: University of Arizona Press.

Chabner, D.E. (2003). *Medical terminology: A short course* (3rd ed.). Philadelphia: W.B. Saunders.

Medical terminology made easy. Available at www.dictionary.com.

Soltesz-Steiner, S. (2003). *Quick medical terminology: A self-teaching guide*. Hoboken, NJ: John Wiley & Sons.

Pharmaceutical and Cosmeceutical Terminology

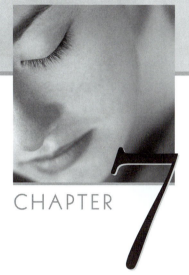

CHAPTER 7

LEARNING OBJECTIVES

After completing this chapter, you should be able to:

1. Discuss the importance of cosmeceutical and pharmaceutical terms in aesthetic skin care.

2. Define how cosmeceutical terms are used.

3. Discuss benefits of the cosmeceutical terminology category.

INTRODUCTION TO COSMECEUTICAL TERMS

The U.S. Food and Drug Administration (FDA) was created in 1938 to review products and keep the citizens of our country safe. The products to be reviewed fell into two categories: (1) the drug (pharmaceuticals) category and (2) a cosmetic (beauty) category. Cosmetics, according to the FDA, are "intended for beautifying and promoting attractiveness."* Drugs, on the other hand, are defined as a "substance used in the diagnosis, cure, and treatment or prevention of disease, *intended to affect the structure and function of the body.*"

---

*Elsner, P., & Maibach, H. L. (Eds.). (2000). *Cosmeceuticals: Drugs vs. cosmetics.* New York: Marcel Dekker.

Cosmeceuticals are found in salons, in medi-spas, on cable shopping networks, and on retail store shelves in varying percentages and pH, making their use (and result) somewhat unpredictable for the average consumer. The opportunities to provide the information necessary to help clients learn to use the product properly vary with the type of retail or service establishment. Pharmaceuticals, on the other hand, are medical in nature and are provided by physician prescription and purchased at pharmacies.

The FDA has not updated or changed the cosmetic or drug categories since its inception, nor does the FDA have any intention to do so in the near future. In many ways, national economics drive the unwillingness of the FDA to change the current laws, as defined in 1938. Chaos would certainly follow if such significant changes were implemented. For example, imagine the uproar if body lotion were to be reclassified as a drug. Although this change is good for cosmetic companies and their products, it does leave room for interpretation as to what constitutes drugs and what constitutes a cosmetic or skin care product. The FDA does not recognize *cosmeceuticals,* and being aware of the term and what it means is important for skin care professionals.

By using the term *cosmeceuticals,* we can differentiate products and create a sense of value for both the clinician and the client. What we would like to achieve with this definition is a categorization of *more-active* products versus those *less-active* products, such as cleansers and moisturizers. Among the products we should classify in this category are alpha hydroxy acids, vitamin C, and retinols. The aforementioned products are not prescriptions but do have scientifically known impact on the skin and its layers. In the medical world of skin care, cosmeceuticals are a staple in the product cabinet. The ingredients are well recognized by clinicians and patients as *active* but not *medicinal.*

The sale of cosmetics is not regulated as rigorously as prescription products that fall under FDA scrutiny. The Federal Food, Drug and Cosmetic (FD&C) Act does not require that cosmetic ingredients undergo approval before they are sold to the public. The FDA does protect the public from harm, however, through packaging requirements. The Fair Packaging and Labeling Act requires that each ingredient appear on the label or be available to consumers. To help the consumer, the ingredients are to appear on the label in descending order of quantity. Additionally, safety testing on cosmetic products is not required. In most instances, however, safety testing is done. If testing is not performed, a warning must appear to that effect: "Warning: The safety of this product has not been determined."

If we were to be purists about both the definition and the potential of products on the skin, we would identify all skin-care products as cosmeceuticals because we know that even a moisturizer will change the barrier effect of the skin.

COSMECEUTICAL AND BOTANICAL DICTIONARY A TO Z

A

abrasive   Also called exfoliate, used to remove loose tissue from body surfaces (e.g., clay, oatmeal powder, rice, pumice, aluminum oxides, salt).

absorbents   Products that break up or disband other substances.

acerola   Shrub having the Barbados cherry that is high in the antioxidant vitamin C.

acetamide MEA   Synthetic material for hair conditioners.

acetic acid   Vinegar; also used as a food preservative.

Aesculus hippocastanum   Horse chestnut, used in toners.

Alchemilla extract   Used for wound healing and antiinflammatory purposes.

alcohol   Organic hydrocarbons with many variations (e.g., absolute, cetyl, dehydrated, denatured, diluted, ethyl, grain isopropyl).

aldehyde   The product that is generated when primary alcohol oxidizes.

algae extract   Considered an active ingredient in skin-care products; improves moisture in the epidermis.

alkaloids   Organic nitrogen-based plant substances.

alkyloamides   Ingredient used in thickening and solubilizing, commonly found in shampoos, liquid hand, and body cleansers.

allantoin   Humectant from comfrey root.

Aloe barbadensis   Aloe vera; nonirritating; may have healing properties.

alpha hydroxy acid   Fruit acids; several variations (e.g., lactic, glycolic, malic).

aluminum   Metallic element used in manufacturing.

aluminosilicates   Components found in clay.

aluminum oxide   Crystal used in microdermabrasion.

ambergris   Used as a fixative; comes from sperm whales.

ammonium laureth sulphate   Surfactant in shampoos, cleansers, and body washes.

ammonium lauryl sulphate   Surfactant; more irritating than ammonium laureth sulphate.

ammonium pareth-25 sulphate   Surfactant used for foaming and cleansing.

Ananas sativus   Pineapple extract; assists with exfoliation of the skin.

anthelmintic   Herb or agent that destroys and dispels worms, parasites, fungus, and yeast from the intestines (e.g., Pau d'arco, goldenseal, wormseed, wormwood, ajwan, cayenne, peppers, pumpkin seeds) (see also vermicide, vermifuge).

antibilious   Herbs that fight nausea and discomfort caused by an over secretion of bile.

antidiarrheal   Herbs that fight diarrhea (e.g., blackberry, red raspberry, ginger).

antiemetic   Herbs that prevent or control nausea and vomiting (e.g., cloves, ginger, raspberry).

antilithic   Herbs that help to prevent stones in the kidney and bladder.

antioxidants   Vitamins and substances that prevent free radical formation (e.g., vitamins A, C, and E).

antiperspirants   Herbs that hamper perspiration.

antiphlogistic   Herbs that help relieve inflammation.

antirheumatic   Herbs that may relieve rheumatism.

antispasmodic   Herbs that assist with muscle spasms or cramps (e.g., chamomile, basil, licorice, sage).

arachidonic acid   Fatty acid.

arachis oil Peanut oil, a carrier substance for skin-care products.

arnica Popular botanical used orally and topically for antiinflammatory and anticoagulant purposes; also used as an antiseptic, astringent, and antimicrobial.

aromatherapy Treatment of mind and body using plant oils and essential oils.

aromatic To have a pleasant fragrance.

ascorbic acid Vitamin C; antioxidant and skin-lightening component.

astringent Topical product used to clarify the skin; restores the natural acidity of the skin.

azulene Antiinflammatory herb found in chamomile.

B

balsam Tree resin for healing and soothing.

barberry extract Has been used for antiseptic and antiinflammatory purposes; also useful for skin eruptions and acne.

barrier cream Creams meant to protect the skin.

bayberry Considered antibacterial; used primarily for acne.

bearberry extract Has astringent and antiseptic properties.

bentonite Nontoxic clay; used in masks and gels.

benzoic acid Preservative especially effective against molds and yeast.

benzoin Essential oil; antibacterial, antiirritant, and antipruritic.

benzophenone Protector against ultraviolet A rays; used in sunscreens.

benzoyl peroxide Bactericidal agent used to treat acne.

benzyl alcohol Preservative effective against bacteria.

beta-carotene From carrot oil; is an antioxidant and has photo protection properties.

beta hydroxy acid Used for treating acne; most common beta hydroxy acid is salicylic acid.

betaines Surfactant that builds viscosity in products; causes foaming.

blackberry extract Used as an astringent, especially for acne.

botanical Pertaining to herbs.

botanical extract Extract of herbs.

bovine From beef.

buffers Chemicals that maintain the pH of an aqueous medium (e.g., sodium bicarbonate).

bulking agent Products used to extend volume (e.g., clays, calcium carbonate, talc).

butylated hydroxyanisole Preservative and antioxidant; not beta hydroxy acid.

butylated hydroxytoluene Antioxidant.

Butyrospermum parkii Shea butter.

C

calamine Mild astringent with cooling qualities used to relive itching.

calcium carbonate Chalk; naturally occurring in limestone, coral, and marble; used in toothpastes and other personal products.

calendula extract (*Calendula officinali*) Herb for treating irritated or inflamed skin; has antiseptic properties (e.g., marigold).

camphor (*Cinnamomum camphora*) Used as anesthetic, antiseptic antiinflammatory agent; also useful as a toner with stringent and cooling properties.

capsicum Herb for circulatory and digestive system (e.g., Spanish pepper).

carageenan Edible seaweed.

carbomer-934 Cross-linked polymer used as a thickener.

carboncysteine Amino acid used for cosmetic preparations.

carboxymethyl cellulose Thickener for bath products and creams.

carminative Herb that helps treat intestinal gas (e.g., chamomile, peppermint).

carmine From the female *Coccu cacti* insect; used for red dye.

carotene Used for a red-orange color in cosmetic formulations.

casein Milk protein used as an emulsifier.

cathartic Related to movement; herbs that evacuate the bowel.

caustic soda (sodium hydroxide) Agent for soap making.

cellulose gum Thickening and stabilizing product.

ceramides Found in cosmetics, assist in the reduction of trans-epidermal water loss (TEWL).

ceteareth-4, -12, -19, -20, -30 Emollient, emulsifier, and lubricant for skin-care products.

cetearyl alcohol Emulsifying wax from plant or natural waxes, used as an emollient.

cetearyl glucoside Emulsifying substance from corn and coconut.

cetrimonium chloride Surfactant used in conditioners; may also be an antiseptic or preservative.

cetyl alcohol Alcohol consisting of mainly n-hexade-canol; used as a thickener and emulsifier (see also cetearyl alcohol).

chamomile Herb that is known to be effective as a bactericidal, antiitching and antiseptic agent; many different types of chamomile plants include German chamomile and Roman chamomile.

chelating agent Agents that enclose a substance to make it inactive.

chelatory agent Substance that binds minerals to itself; in cosmetic manufacture, refers to chemicals that mop up free ions, such as metals, in formulae and inhibit them from causing deterioration of the product.

chlorophyll Natural coloring agent; may smooth and heal the skin.

chloroxethanol Preservative.

cholagogue Herb that improves the flow of bile (e.g., licorice, safflower, senna).

Chondrus crispus Seaweed.

Cinnamonum zeylanicum Cinnamon oil said to be antimicrobial and antiseptic.

citric acid Antioxidant and astringent; from citrus fruits.

Citrus bergamia Herb with antiseptic properties (e.g., bergamot orange essential oil).

Citrus grandis Grape seed oil; has possible antiseptic properties.

citrus paradisi Grapefruit essential oil; an astringent and antiseptic; rich in vitamin C; from the seeds of grapefruit.

clay Used in liquids, creams, and facemasks; varieties could include bentonite, beetum, and kaotin.

coal tar Used in antidandruff shampoos.

cocamide diethanolamide Increases viscosity for surfactant systems; used in liquid cleansers.

cocamidopropyi betaine Properly called cocamidopropyi dimethyl glycine; a member of the betaine family used as a mild foaming and cleansing agent to reduce the irritancy of harsher surfactants in shampoos.

cocamonium carbamoylchloride Foaming surfactant with thickening properties.

cocos nucifera Coconut oil; emollient uses.

coemulsifiers Emulsifiers added to product to stabilize the product systems.

collagen Found in skin, cartilage, and other connective tissues; gives the skin support and a youthful appearance.

color additive Products used to add color to skin care products; iron oxides.

comedogenic Cosmetics or products that cause the skin to become congested and form acne pustules.

comfrey extract Used as a healing agent; also has emollient properties.

Commiphore myrrha Antiseptic, antimicrobial, antiinflammatory; from the Myrrh bush.

contact dermatitis Treats inflammation of the skin (e.g., redness, rash, itching).

copper Nontoxic, as a trace element in topical preparations; has a catalytic action for keratinization; may also play a role in the formation of collagen by promoting certain enzymatic activities.

cosmeceutical Products with active ingredients; usually found in physician offices or medical spas.

D

dandelion extract   Herb that is rich in minerals; used as a topical tonic to correct pH.

daucus carota   Herb that has antioxidant properties; precursor to vitamin A.

decyl alcohol   Antifoaming agent.

decyl glucoside   Foaming agent.

decyl polyglucose   Used in cleansers for its foaming factor.

demulcent   Herb that acts on the mucous membranes (e.g., barley, licorice, linseed).

deodorant   Masks the bacterial odor of perspiration.

depilatory   Cream used to remove hair.

depurative   Herb to purify the blood.

detergent (foaming agent)   Used to foam and cleanse using a surfactant.

diaphoretic   Promotes perspiration (e.g., juniper berries, barley, chamomile, dandelion, spearmint).

diatomaceous earth   An abrasive agent for cleansers and exfoliates.

diethanolamine   Organic alkali used to neutralize organic acids.

digestives   Herbs that assist with digestion (e.g., cumin, turmeric).

dimethicone   From silicone; used for lubrication in skin care products.

dioctyl sodium sulfosuccinate   Surfactant.

disinfectant   Destroys germs; could be herbal or chemical.

disodium EDTA (ethylenediamine tetra-acetic acid)   Preservative.

DMDM (3'-Demethoxy-3o-Demethylmatai-resinol) hydantoin   Safe, widely used preservative.

E

Echinacea   Has antibacterial properties; seems to shorten the healing time of skin lesions.

EDTA   Ethylenediamine tetra-acetic acid; augments a formulations preservative system.

elastin   Found in cosmetic preparations; used topically for the purpose of moisturizing. Related to collagen.

Eleais guineensis   Palm kernel oil; an emollient and lubricant.

electrolyte   Used to thicken cosmetics and shampoos (e.g., salt).

emetic   Causes vomiting.

emollient   Topical cosmetic preparation to help promote smoothness and flexibility of the skin.

emulsifier   Reduces surface tension; used in cosmetic preparations to bind soluble oil and water ingredients.

emulsion   Mixture of soluble oil and water ingredients found in most creams and lotions.

emulsion stabilizer   Assists with the formation and stabilization of cosmetic creams and lotions.

enzyme   An organic catalyst produced by cells to create chemical reactions; digestive enzymes break up food and synthesize proteins for body use.

epsom salts   Magnesium sulphate used for detoxifying.

essential fatty acid   Fatty acid that cannot be supplied by the body; must be part of the diet.

essential oil   Botanic origins achieved through steam distillation or mechanical expression; used therapeutically at home or in the clinic or spa.

ester   From an acid; may have a fruity smell.

ethanol   Alcohol.

ethyl alcohol   Rubbing alcohol.

Eucalyptus oil   Antiseptic and disinfectant; used originally by the Aborigines; may cause allergic responses.

exfoliate   Removes surface dead skin cells with the use of an abrasive agent; found in synthetic or natural grains.

expression   Technique used for extracting the essential oils from citrus products.

F

farnesol   Bioactivator; a component of vitamin K; found in lilac, lily of the valley, and sandalwood.

fennel extract Antiseptic and detoxifier; used for oily skin.

fluoride Inorganic substance added to toothpaste to prevent decay.

formula Recipe but expressed in percentages rather than weights and measurements.

fructose Naturally occurring sugar.

fungicide Product that kills fungi.

fungistatic Inhibits the growth of fungi.

G

G Gram; a measurement.

glucose glutamate Humectant used in hand creams and lotions.

glycerin Popular humectant used in moisturizers; binds water.

glycerin monostearate Popular for creams; functions as emulsifying agent and solubilizing agent.

glycoceramides May replace lost intercorneal lipids; helps the skin bind water.

glycocitrates Combination of glycolic acid and citric acids; meant for skin that is sensitive or unable to tolerate glycolic acids.

glycolic acid Solution for use in gels, creams, and peel solutions; has exfoliating properties.

glycosaminoglycans Polysaccharides; help the skin retain and hold water; used in cosmetic moisturizing preparations.

glycyrrhizic acid From licorice root; has antibacterial properties.

GRAS Generally recognized as safe.

guar hydroxypropyltrimonium chloride Antiinflammatory and antiirritant; may have skin-softening capabilities.

H

Hamamelis virginia Witch hazel; astringent.

hectorite Thickening agent.

homomenthyl salicylate Component of some sunscreens; absorbs ultraviolet B rays.

humectant Agent for retaining moisture.

hyaluronic acid Component of glycosaminoglycans; a natural component of the skin.

hydrogen peroxide Antiseptic agent.

hydrolysis Common process whereby water and a salt produce a product with an acid and a base; a common occurrence of during conversion of protein to amino acids in the digestive process.

hydrolyzed mucopolysaccharides Has properties that assist in treating TEWL; produced from animal polysaccharides.

I

imidazolidinyl urea Antimicrobial agent, antibacterial preservative; commonly used.

ingredient list List of product composition by weight.

insoluble Does not dissolve.

iron oxide Pigment for cosmetics.

isocetyl stearate Emollient.

isodecyl oleate Emollient and wetting agent; also binds pigment.

isoluitane Propellant used in aerosol products.

isopropyl palmitate From coconut oil; an emollient and moisturizer.

J

No entries

K

kaolin Aluminum silicate; used in masks and powders.

KG Kilogram.

KOH (potassium hydroxide) Caustic potash-potassium lye.

L

L Liter.

lactic acid Alpha hydroxy acid used in skin-care products as an emollient, moisturizer, and preservative.

laneth-10 For emulsifying lanolin.

lanolin Emollient; high water-inclusion properties; a controversial product given that studies show low incidence of allergy or irritation; derived from sheep wool.

lanolin alcohol Emollient and emulsifier used in water-in-oil systems.

lapsana Antioxidant; protective for the skin.

lauramide Stabilizes foam; builds viscosity.

laureth-1 to -23 Has emulsifying properties.

lauric acid Stabilizes foam.

lauryl alcohol Skin conditioner, emollient.

lauryl lysine Amino acid; used as a skin conditioner.

***Lavandula angustifolia* (lavender essential oil)** Used for its calming and healing properties; a good choice for sensitive skin.

lecithin Emulsifier and antioxidant found in soybeans and eggs for cosmetic use.

linoleic acid Emulsifier; improves dry skin.

linoleic acid triglyceride Good emollient that penetrates well but goes bad in the product quickly.

liposomes Phospholipid delivery device for skin-care products.

lysine Amino acid for skin conditioning.

M

magnesium Important in enzyme reactions; contributes to amino acid synthesis.

magnesium aluminum silicate Thickener.

malic acid Alpha hydroxy acid; found in apples.

Melaleuca alternifolia Tea tree essential oil; popular for use as an antiseptic.

methicone Silicone used in cosmetic powders.

mica Creates the glitter in eye shadow.

mineral oil Good in cleansers; comedogenicity depends on the level of product refinement.

mucopolysaccharide Reduces TEWL; binds to water.

mud Powder and liquid; used as masks for the treatment of congested skin.

myristic acid Cleansing agent works especially well when combine with potassium.

myristyl alcohol Emollient; used in hand creams.

N

natural Describes subjectively the idea that the products are not synthetic but come from nature; not a dependable term and should not be the only qualifier for selection of a product.

natural coloring Unprocessed cosmetic dyes; less toxic but more likely to fade.

niacin Vitamin B3.

niacinamide Vitamin B3.

nonionic surfactant Agent without an electric charge.

Nymphaea alba Water lily extract; soothing and calming for the skin.

O

occlusive agent Product that prevents the skin from breathing (e.g., Vaseline®).

octocrylene Water-resistant sunscreen agent; protects against ultraviolet B rays.

octyl salicylate Sunscreen; noncomedogenic.

Oenothera biennis Evening primrose essential oil; used for dry skin.

oil Natural hydrocarbon found in plants, animals, and minerals.

ointment base Product ingredient added to an ointment (e.g., steroids).

olea europaea Olive oil; emollient and lubricant.

oleic acid Emollient; has skin-penetrating properties.

oligoelement Trace elements.

opacifying agent Substance added to create opaque colors.

P

PABA (paraaminobenzoic acid) Water-soluble acid in B vitamins; used as sunscreen; can cause irritation.

panthenol Vitamin B5; moisturizer.

papain   Papaya enzyme found in pineapples; used as an exfoliate.

parabens   Most common preservatives in cosmetic products.

paraffin wax   Wax used for moisturizers and thickening.

pectin   Thickener for cosmetics.

PEG derivatives -4, -8, -14, -20, -32, -75, -100, -150, -200 (polyethylene glycol)   Numbers represent weight; used for product consistency, spreadability, moisture resistance, or oxidation resistance.

Pelargonium graveolens   Geranium essential oil; used in toners.

pentasodium pentate   Emulsifier and agent for dissolving moisturizers.

Persea gratissima   Avocado essential oil; used as an emollient; excellent for dry skin.

petroleum jelly   Lubricant and emollient; an occlusive agent.

phenol   Organic acid; powerful peel solution.

phenoxyethanol   Antimicrobial agent used with parabens.

phenyl dimethicone   Inhibits foaming.

phosphoric acid   Used to adjust product pH.

phytotherapy   Treatment using plants and herbs used for therapeutic value.

p-isoamyi methoxycinnamate   Ultraviolet ray filter.

polyacrylamide   Polymer used as a thickener in tanning products.

polymer   Substance that combines small molecules.

potassium sulfate   Product to increase viscosity in cosmetics.

poultice   Plant material applied to the surface of the body as a remedy.

propolis   From bees wax; a sunlight protective agent; also used for acne care.

propyl parabens   Low-sensitivity, low-toxicity preservative.

propylene glycol   Solvent, humectant, and moisturizing agent. Common water-carrying vehicle in cosmetics; well received by the skin.

pseudocollagen   From plants; acts as a moisturizing film on the skin.

pyruvic acid   Alpha hydroxy acid derived from sodium pyruvate; has a large molecule.

Q

No entries

R

retinyl esters   Products that are precursors to retinoic acid.

retinyl palmitate   Substance used for conditioning the skin; milder than retinoic acid.

riboflavin (vitamin B)   Emollient in skin-care products.

S

saccharide   Moisturizing agent.

salicylic acid   Used as a peel solution; has a strong keratolytic activity; digests the debris in follicles; good for treating acne.

Santalum alba   Sandalwood essential oil; used for dry, dehydrated skin.

saponins   Substances that create foam when shaken.

SD alcohol   Denatured alcohol for cosmetic use.

seaweed extract   From one of the many varieties of seaweed; has strong healing properties.

silicone   Stable component for use in facial creams; prevents water evaporation from the skin.

sodium benzoate   Antiseptic and preservative for cosmetics.

sodium bicarbonate   Alkaline substance; used to adjust skin pH in peeling or in skin-care products.

sodium chloride   Astringent; also a thickener (common table salt).

sodium lauryl sulphate   Synthetic detergent commonly used in shampoos and cleansers.

sodium silicate   Component found in clays (e.g., kaolin, bentonite).

sorbic acid   Humectant and preservative.

sorbitol   Humectant and binding agent.

SPF   Sun protection factor; indicates the level of protection against harmful sunlight.

squalene   From shark liver oil; lubricant, compatible with human skin.

steareth compounds   Solubilizers and coemulsifiers.

stearic acid   Emulsifier and thickener; produced from vegetable fats.

styptic   Astringent; controls bleeding (e.g., styptic pencil).

sunscreens   Substances to protect the skin from the sun's burning rays.

T

tallow   Occlusive to the skin; primary agent in soaps; cultivated from animal fatty tissue.

tannins   Astringents.

tartaric acid   Alpha hydroxy acid; not frequently used.

TEA (triethanolamine)   Emulsifier.

terpinol   Active ingredient of tea tree essential oil.

tetrasodium   Preservative and chelating agent.

thickener   Ingredient used to improve the solidity or viscosity of a product.

tincture   Herb prepared with alcohol and water.

titanium dioxide   Nonchemical substance that acts as a physical sun block.

tocopherol   Vitamin E.

triclosan   Preservative.

Triticum vulgare   Wheat germ essential oil.

tyrosine   Amino acid; topical applications stimulate melanin synthesis.

U

urea   Increases the absorption of product ingredients.

USP   *United States Pharmacopoeia.*

V

vegetable oil   Oil from a plant.

vitamin A   Necessary for the regeneration of skin cells; vitamin A esters convert to retinoic acid in the skin. Vitamin A improves the skin's tone, texture and density.

vitamin B   Currently controversial as to how or if vitamin B can penetrate the skin surface.

vitamin C   Known antioxidant that improves the skin's tone and texture; also has some minor solar protection properties.

vitamin D   Vital to the epidermal process; seems to improve the tone and texture of the skin.

vitamin E   Antioxidant.

vitamin E acetate   Free-radical scavenger; very stable.

vitamin E linoleate   Synthetic vitamin E.

vitamin F   Linoleic acid; used to treat dry skin.

vitamin H   Biotin; for treating acne.

vitamin P   Possible protection of collagen destruction.

W

wax   Water-repellent esters.

W/O   Water in oil (emulsion).

X

xanthan gum   Polysaccharide produced from bacteria; used as a thickener, emulsifier, and stabilizer.

xyloglucan   Extract from plants; antiseptic in nature.

Y

No entries

Z

zinc oxide   Has antimicrobial, preservative, and water-resistant capabilities; popular for use in sunscreens.

EXERCISES

Part A

Define the following terms:

1. abrasive _____

   _____

2. absorbents _____

   _____

3. acetic acid _____

   _____

4. aluminum oxide _____

   _____

5. ammonium laureth sulphate _____

   _____

6. ammonium lauryl sulphate _____

   _____

7. antioxidants _____

   _____

8. aromatic _____

   _____

9. ascorbic acid _____

   _____

10. astringent _____

    _____

11. balsam _____

    _____

12. benzoic acid _____

    _____

13. benzyol peroxide _____

    _____

14. benzyl alcohol _____

    _____

15. beta-carotene _____

    _____

16. botanical _____

    _____

17. calamine _____

    _____

18. calcium carbonate _____

    _____

19. carotene _____

    _____

20. ceramides _____

    _____

Continued

EXERCISES

Part A—cont'd

Define the following terms:

21. citric acid _____

_____

22. cocamidopropyi betaine _____

_____

23. collagen _____

_____

24. copper _____

_____

25. depurative _____

_____

26. Echinacea _____

_____

27. elastin _____

_____

28. emollient _____

_____

29. emulsifier _____

_____

30. enzyme _____

_____

31. fluoride _____

_____

32. fungicide _____

_____

33. glycerin _____

_____

34. humectant _____

_____

35. hyaluronic acid _____

_____

36. hydrolysis _____

_____

37. isopropyl palmitate _____

_____

38. lactic acid _____

_____

39. liposomes _____

_____

40. magnesium _____

_____

EXERCISES

Part A—cont'd

Define the following terms:

41. methicone _____

42. niacin _____

43. niacinamide _____

44. PABA _____

45. panthenol _____

46. papain _____

47. petroleum jelly _____

48. phenol _____

49. phosphoric acid _____

50. pyruvic acid _____

51. retinyl palmitate _____

52. salicylic acid _____

53. sodium lauryl sulphate _____

54. titanium dioxide _____

55. xanthan gum _____

INTRODUCTION TO PHARMACEUTICAL TERMS

Pharmaceutical products are drugs or products that heal or prevent disease. According to the FDA, the definition of these products are "substances used in the diagnosis, cure, and treatment or prevention of disease;

*intended to affect the structure and function of the body."** We think of drugs as antibiotics, prescription pain medications, or products that correct a disease process such as diabetes, high blood pressure, and epilepsy. However, some pharmaceutical products are both *drugs* and *cosmetics* (e.g., sunscreens, dandruff shampoos). This classification is a result of the active ingredients found in these items. The FDA requires that these products list the active ingredients first followed by the remaining ingredients in descending order.

PHARMACEUTICAL TERMS A TO Z

A

acetone   Noncomedogenic occasionally used in toners and nail-polish removers; used to prep skin before a chemical peel.

acid   Substances with a low pH value; has irritating properties.

active ingredient   Ingredients that cause improvement or action.

ADR   Adverse drug reaction.

adverse reaction   Undesirable effects or toxicity.

aerobic   Living only with oxygen.

agar   Gel unaffected by bacterial enzymes; used as culture medium.

agglutination   Antigen-antibody reaction; sticking together of cells; occurs when the wrong blood type is transfused.

albumin   Group of simple proteins; egg whites.

alkalinity   Increase in base bicarbonate; the opposite of acidity.

allergenic extract   Substance that creates an allergic response.

amino acids   Proteins.

ampholyte   Behaves as an acid or a base.

amphoteric   Characteristics of opposites.

anabolism   Productive phase of metabolism; the opposite of catabolism.

Anaerobe   Living with oxygen.

analgesic   Pain reliever.

ancillary material   Used to prepare drugs; not a component of the drug.

anesthetics   Loss of sensation.

anion   Negatively charged particle or ion.

antibacterial   Inhibits the increase and duplicate of bacteria.

antibiotic   Toxic to or inhibiting to microbial organisms; to fight infection.

antibody   Glycoprotein associated with gamma globulin; produced to fight infections or disease.

antielastase   Slows down the action of elastase.

antigen   Marker on the cell that defines the type (e.g., skin, liver, kidney); markers stimulate antibodies.

antipyretic   Drug that reduces fever.

antiseptic   Used to decontaminate surfaces and objects; inhibits the growth of bacteria.

antitoxin   Used in response to biologic toxins (e.g., tetanus).

ascomycetes   True fungi (e.g., yeast, molds).

asepsis   Disease producing organisms are not present.

auto immune disease   Body's antigenic markers disappear creating a disease (e.g., lupus).

---

*Pharmaceuticals are subject to FDA approval, a long and arduous process that can take years to complete. Furthermore, drugs are manufactured by specific companies that have many regulations and processes in place to meet the requirements of the FDA rules.

autoclave   Machine that provides moist heat sterilization.

avobenzone (BMDM [butyl methoxydiben-zoylmethane])   Chemical sunscreen agent, works on ultraviolet A rays.

B

bactericide   Destroys bacteria but not its spores.

bacteriostatic   Slows the growth of bacterial organisms.

bacterium   One-celled organism; round, rod-shaped, spiral or filamentous in nature.

biochemistry   Chemical study of living beings.

biocide   Kills all organisms.

biodegradable   Biologic action that breaks down materials.

biohazard   Dangerous to humans, plants, and animals.

biologic   From living beings.

biopsy   Section of tissue taken for examination, gross and microscopic.

blood plasma   Blood in which only platelet cells remain; a clear, straw-colored fluid.

blood platelets   Component of blood; essential for clotting.

bloodborne pathogens   Found in human or animal blood that carries infectious microorganisms that can be transmitted to others through contact with blood, body fluids, and other forms of contact.

broad spectrum   Wide range.

BTU (British thermal unit)   To measure heat.

C

C   Celsius; temperature scale; also known as centigrade.

calcium   Metallic element; chemical symbol Ca.

calibration   Process used to ensure a machine's accuracy; to calibrate.

calorie   Measurement of heat.

carbohydrates   Nutrient required by the body; one of six.

carcinogen   Substance that causes cancerous growths.

carrier   Has a specific pathogenic organism or mutated gene; the substance in which a topical product may float.

catalyst   Substance that increases the rate of reaction.

cation   Positively charged particle.

cell   Component that is the basis of life.

centrifuge   Device used to spin liquids or blood into two separate solutions (e.g., solids, liquids).

chelating   Agents to grip a substance and make it inactive.

chemotherapy   Treatment of disease by chemical means.

chlorine   An element used to disinfect water.

chromosome   Genetic structure; cells of DNA.

clone   Genetically identical cells.

clostridium   Bacteria; anaerobic spore-forming rod.

coagulation   To clump together.

coccus   Bacteria; round or sphere like.

coenzyme   Molecule that is needed for certain enzyme actions; many times has a vitamin attached.

collagen   Protein found in connective tissue; many different types.

compounding   Putting together components to create products; usually active ingredients.

contaminant   Undesired component in a controlled environment.

contamination   The process of bringing undesired components.

cross-contamination   Undesirable result of components that move to another material (e.g., from one jar of product into another jar of product).

culture medium   Mixture of organic and inorganic product used to grow bacteria or other cells.

cytokine   Protein that acts as a chemical messenger.

cytoplasm   Contents outside the cell nucleus; where the organelles are suspended.

cytotoxic   Poisonous to cells.

D

decontamination   Process to reduce contaminating substances.

diagnostic   Serving to understand or identify a disease or problem.

dilution   Process of lowering of the concentration.

diploid   Paired chromosomes; 46 pairs for humans.

disinfection   Process of reducing microbiological agents to reduce disease.

diuretic   Product or drug to increase urination.

DNA   Deoxyribonucleic acid; molecular base for genes; contains inherited characteristics.

dosage form   How a drug is delivered (e.g., topical, tablet).

double-blind test   Used for clinical trials of a product in which parties are unaware of whether the product is a placebo or the actual product until the end of testing.

drugs   Products for the cure and treatment of disease or health problems.

dry heat sterilization   Sterilization in an oven, not in an autoclave.

durability   Wherewithal to withstand a rigorous test.

dynamic conditions   Constant change.

E

efficacy   How well a product or treatment works or achieves the desired result.

elastin   Protein connective tissue, usually found in the middle layer of arteries.

electrolyte   Compound dissolved in a solution and conducts a current of electricity.

endocrine glands   Glands that secrete hormones that are carried (via blood) to specific organs (e.g., pituitary, pancreas, ovaries, testes).

endorphins   Polypeptide produced by the brain; creates analgesia.

endospore   Thick-walled spore.

endotoxin   Poisonous molecule that is part of gram-negative bacteria.

enzyme   Protein that promotes reactions.

epithelium   Layer of cells.

erythrocyte   Red blood cell manufactured in the bone marrow; has oxygen-carrying hemoglobin.

Escherichia coli (E. coli)   Gram-negative bacteria; fast growing; commonly found in the gastrointestinal (GI) tract; usually causes infections outside the GI tract.

essential amino   Substance necessary for human life but must be consumed in the diet.

etiologic agent   Organism that causes disease.

exanthematous   Skin eruption (e.g., measles, fever blisters).

exotoxins   Toxic substance created by microorganisms and released into surrounding tissue.

expiration date   Date after which a product or drug should not be used; end of product life expectancy.

F

F   Fahrenheit; temperature measurement.

fatty acid   Monobasic acid important for maintaining a healthy skin; excellent as emollients.

FDA   U.S. Food and Drug Administration.

fibrin   Plasma protein.

fibrinogen   Component of the blood clotting process.

folic acid   Component of vitamin B complex.

follicle   Small anatomic cavity containing the hair root and sweat gland.

formaldehyde   Colorless, pungent gas used as a antimicrobial agent.

free radicals   Unpaired ions.

fungi   Plural of fungus.

fungicide   Agent that destroys fungi.

G

gel   Semisolid (colloidal) substance; contains large amounts of water.

gene   Unit of hereditary; contains DNA.

generic drug   Product made and advertised under the chemical name.

genetic diseases   Diseases that occur in genetic material.

genetic engineering   Process of changing the genes by technologic means.

genetics   Study of heredity: how particular qualities or traits are transmitted.

germicidal lamp   Device that emits ultraviolet radiation that kills bacteria, viruses, and fungi.

germicide   Agent that destroys microorganisms or germs.

Golgi bodies   Small particles responsible for some enzyme secretion.

H

harvesting   Process of separating cells.

hazardous substance   Agent that is dangerous (i.e., flammable, toxic, poisonous).

health hazard   Event or substance in which exposure may cause chronic health problems (e.g., cancer, damage to body systems).

heat   Form of energy.

helix   Conformation of biologic polymers.

hemoglobin   Red blood cells.

hemopoietic   Relate to describing or making blood cells.

heparin   Polysaccharide that prevents the blood from clotting.

hepatotoxin   Agent that is destructive to the liver cells.

heterotrophs   Organism requiring complex foods (e.g., carbohydrates or lipids to grow and develop).

histamine   Chemical released via the body's immune system in response to allergens.

hormone   Messenger to inhibit or stimulate metabolic activities.

human gene therapy   Form of treatment by inserting DNA into cells to correct a genetic defect.

human genome   Full collection of genes for human reproduction.

hydrocarbon   A molecule that is hydrogen and carbon; usually found as propellants in aerosols.

hydroquinone   Bleaching agent for the skin.

hygienic   Related to the concept of being clean.

hypnotic   Tendency to produce sleep.

hypoallergenic   Without fragrance (in the strictest sense); more broadly refers to products that are unlikely to cause skin irritation.

I

immunity   State of being protected from disease by having been exposed to the antigen marker.

immunology   Study of the body's defense against disease.

inactive ingredient   Agent that does not function actively.

inert   Lacking in the ability to dissolve in water or react with other substances chemically.

infarct   An area of tissue that becomes necrotic resulting from failure of the blood supply.

infected   Contaminated with tissue-damaging microorganisms.

innocuous   Noncontaminated.

ionic   Relating to ions.

irritant   Any agent that reacts on the skin creating inflammation.

isotretinoin   Agent used to treat acne using a keratolytic action.

K

keratin   Protein substance found in hair and nails.

keratolytic   Agent that causes the skin to shed.

L

lipid   Substance that is fatlike and is not soluble in water.

lipoprotein   Bond of a simple protein and a lipid (e.g., cholesterol).

liposome   Vesicle formed when particular lipids are added to a water-based solution, creating a seal that encapsulates the solution; can be used to slowly release a drug into the body.

lymphocyte   Type of white blood cell that occurs before the formation of antibodies.

lysis   Gradual decline or the process of breaking apart.

lysosome   Cell organelle that contain hydrolytic enzymes that help digest proteins and carbohydrates internally.

M

macrophage   Cell of the immune system, recruited to remove debris after injury.

medicated products   Products with ingredients to sooth.

melanin   Pigment of the skin, hair, and eyes.

melanoma   Most aggressive skin cancer; originates at melanocytes.

membrane   Thin barrier.

metabolism   Physical and chemical changes in the cell.

metastasis   Spread of a disease (e.g., cancer).

milliequivalent   Chemical equivalent; one thousandth.

mitosis   Cell division.

mL   Milliliter.

molds   Growth of fungus on a surface; fuzzy.

molecular weight   Molecule's weight.

monosaccharide   Simple sugar, carbohydrates; building blocks.

MSDS (material safety data sheet)   Safety sheet for substances.

mucous membranes   Tissue linings in the respiratory and genitourinary tracts.

multicellular   More than one cell.

N

narcotic   Addicting substance that reduces pain and produces sleep.

necrosis   Irreversible death of cells and as such tissue.

normal saline   Solution used to mix drugs or irrigate wounds.

nucleic acid   Nucleotide subunits.

nucleus   Component of the cell that contains genetic material; a cellular organelle.

O

ophthalmic   Pertaining to the eye.

ophthalmics   Area of health care pertaining to the eyes.

organelles   Found in eukaryotic cells; contain enzymes and other material necessary for cell function.

organic   Natural and human-made molecules.

organism   Living being.

osmosis   Diffusion of a solvent through a membrane, which changes the concentrations when the solution moves through.

oxidation   Reaction involving oxygen.

P

pandemic disease   Disease over a wide geographic region.

patch test   Test to measure a drug or treatment on a small patch of skin to determine the suitability of the product or treatment.

permeability   State of being able to pass a fluid under pressure.

permeate   To diffuse through or penetrate something (e.g., reverse osmosis).

pH   Describes acidity or alkalinity.

pharmaceutical   Drug or medicine to treat disease or illness.

plasma   Liquid of blood and lymph.

poison   Substance dangerous to life.

polypeptide   Chain of amino acids.

potent Strong and active, usually pertaining to a substance.

precipitate Suspension that separates from a solution.

preservative Agent added to keep bacteria from a food or drug to prevent spoilage.

prophylaxis Preventative treatment.

protease Protein that can divide other proteins.

protein Amino acid necessary for growth and development.

proteolysis Hydrolysis of protein; destruction of protein.

protoplasm Thick fluid that is the basis for all life.

protozoa Microorganisms; smallest organisms known.

purification Process of removing impurities.

solvent Agent used to prepare solutions or suspension.

spore Beginning of algae or fungi.

sporicide Agent that kills bacterial and fungal spores.

stability Ability to remain unchanged; number of years a product is good before it should be discarded.

starch Sugar polymer; used in cosmetics for its absorbency.

sterilization Process of destroying bacteria, fungi, and spores.

substrate Substance on which enzymes react.

surfactant Agent that reduces the surface tension of a product; allows product to function better.

suspension Particles mixed in a liquid.

synthesis Process of creating (e.g., chemical and enzyme reactions).

R

resorcinol Type of peel solution; a component of Jessner peel solutions.

retinoids Topical vitamin A.

S

salmonella Gram-negative rod; causes food poisoning in humans.

sanitization Decontamination that decreases microorganisms.

sepsis Pus-forming pathogenic organisms in the blood (e.g., septicemia).

sodium lactate Liquid that assists in keeping the skin's pH more alkaline; produces moisture binding.

solute Dissolved substance (e.g., ions) to form a solution.

solublizer Agent that assists in breaking down nonsoluble products or ingredients.

T

temperature Heat or cold measurement.

terminal sterilization Process whereby something goes from nonsterile to sterile.

terminally ill State of illness that will cause a patient to die.

thrombosis Clotting.

titration Addition of small amounts until the desired concentration is met.

topical product Medication applied to the skin.

toxicology The science of poisons.

toxin Poisonous agent.

tumor Growth of abnormal cells.

tyrosine Triiodothyronine; also related to the black pigment melanin.

V

viscosity Property of resistance to flow (i.e., pourability, stickiness).

W

wetting agent Substance that increases the spreading of a liquid by reducing the tension between two surfaces.

white blood cell Blood cell without the oxygen carrying components of a red blood cell.

X

X chromosome Sex chromosome; female.

Y

Y chromosome Sex chromosome; male.

yeasts Unicellular fungi.

Common Medical Abbreviations from Latin

Abbreviation	Meaning	Latin
ad lib	freely as wanted	*ad libitum*
aq.	water	*aqua*
bid	twice a day	*bis in die*
c (with bar on top)	with	*cum*
cap	capsule	*capula*
eq pts	equal parts	*equalis partis*
gtt	a drop	*gutta*
h	hour	*hora*
no	number	*numero*
prn	as occasion requires	*pro re nata*
qd	every day	*quaque 1 die*
q4h	every 4 hours	*quaque 4 hora*
q6h	every 6 hours	*quaque 6 hora*
qid	four times a day	*quater in die*
qsqd	a sufficient quantity every day	*quantum sufficiatquaque 1 die*
qw	every week	
sid	once a day	*semel in die*
Sig, S	write on the label	*signa*
stat	immediately	*statim*
tab	a tablet	*tabella*
tid	three times a day	*ter in die*

EXERCISES

Part B

Fill in the blanks.

1. Topical vitamin A is a _____.

2. *gtts* means _____.

3. The pigment of the skin is created by _____.

4. Synthesis is to _____.

5. Preventative treatment is called _____.

6. The science of poisons is _____.

7. Oxidation is _____.

8. A polypeptide produced by the brain that creates analgesia is _____.

9. An organism that is living without oxygen is _____.

10. A product that kills bacterial and fungal spores is called _____.

11. The bond of a simple protein and a lipid (e.g., cholesterol) is _____.

12. An undesired component in a controlled environment is called _____.

13. The most aggressive skin cancer is called _____.

14. A protein substance found in hair and nails is called _____.

15. *tid* means _____.

16. *prn* means _____.

17. An undesirable effect or toxicity is _____.

18. An addicting substance that reduces pain and produces sleep is called a _____.

19. A messenger to inhibit or stimulate metabolic activities is called _____.

Continued

EXERCISES

Part B—cont'd

Fill in the blanks.

20. A compound dissolved in a solution that conducts a current of electricity is called _____.

21. The process of bringing undesired components is called _____.

22. A machine used to spin liquids or blood into two separate solutions (e.g., solids and liquids) is called

    _____.

23. A measurement of heat is called _____.

24. Disease over a wide geographic region is referred to as _____.

25. Glands that secrete hormones that are carried (via blood) to specific organs are called

    _____.

CONCLUSION

A complete understanding of pharmaceutical and cosmeceutical terms is critical to the education of the future aesthetician. Remembering all of these terms is difficult, and this chapter is meant to serve as a reference guide to help you remember these terms. Cosmeceuticals and pharmaceuticals have an effect on the skin and on the skin's condition. To be the most effective practitioner of the art of aesthetics, it is equally important to be familiar with not only the active ingredients, but also with the inactive ingredients and terms associated with the products that you use and recommend to your clients.

CHAPTER REFERENCE

Elsner, P., & Maibach, H. L. (Eds.). (2000). *Cosmeceuticals: Drugs vs. cosmetics*. New York: Marcel Dekker.

Answer Key

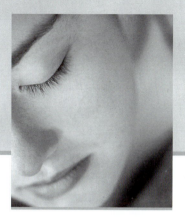

Chapter 3

Part A
1. CARCIN/O/GEN
2. LAPAR/O/SCOPY
3. ADEN/OMA
4. ARTHR/ITIS
5. BI/O/LOGY
6. CEPH/A/LIC
7. CYT/O/LOGY
8. ELECTR/O/ CARDI/O/GRAM
9. ENTER/O/LOGY
10. HEMA/A/TOMA
11. LEUK/O/CYTE
12. REN/AL
13. PATH/O/GEN
14. NEUR/AL
15. PSYCH/O/SIS
16. RHIN/O/PLASTY
17. SAR/COMA

Part B
1. stomach
2. cancer
3. abdomen
4. gland
5. joints
6. life

7. head
8. cell
9. electric
10. intestine
11. blood
12. white
13. kidney
14. disease
15. brain
16. mind
17. nose
18. flesh

Part C
1. pertaining to the stomach
2. producing cancer
3. to view the abdomen
4. abdominal tumor
5. inflammation of the joints
6. the study of life
7. pertaining to the head
8. the study of cells
9. device used to record electric activity of the heart
10. the study of intestines
11. cancer of the blood

12. white blood cells
13. pertaining to the kidney
14. producing disease
15. pertaining to the brain
16. state of mind considered to be unhealthy
17. formation of the nose
18. tumor of the flesh

Part D
1. a
2. x
3. en
4. ex
5. is
6. um
7. us
8. y
9. oma

Part E
1. indices
2. thoraces
3. deformities
4. ganglia
5. carcinomata
6. patellea

Part E—cont'd
7. ova
8. lumina
9. diagnoses

Part F
1. dysphagia
2. prognastism
3. phrenoplegia
4. cochlea
5. hemoptysis
6. polypnea
7. gnathitis
8. dysanthia
9. pneumonic
10. haema
11. pneometer
12. rugae
13. rhytidosis
14. coelum
15. psoriasis
16. septicaemia
17. pterygoid
18. xanthic

Chapter 4
Part A
1. port
2. decis
3. dict
4. gno
5. cephal
6. dict
7. port

Part B
1. r
2. b
3. e
4. c
5. s
6. f
7. t
8. h
9. u
10. d
11. j
12. k
13. o
14. v
15. w
16. l
17. p
18. m
19. q
20. i

Part C
1. extremities
2. gland
3. elbow
4. cavity
5. joint
6. eyelid
7. airway
8. heart
9. wrist
10. head
11. lip
12. hand
13. colon
14. cranium
15. bladder
16. cell
17. digit
18. skin
19. ligaments
20. testicle
21. tongue
22. blood
23. liver
24. tissue
25. uterus
26. hip
27. horny tissue
28. abdomen
29. larynx
30. fat
31. breast
32. limbs
33. spinal cord
34. muscle
35. kidney
36. nerve
37. tooth
38. eye
39. bone
40. ear
41. vein
42. foot
43. rectum
44. nose
45. pulse
46. chest
47. nipple
48. neck
49. hair

Part D
1. ac
2. vari
3. tum
4. adi
5. alveol
6. alb
7. annul
8. apic
9. aqu
10. articul
11. string
12. are
13. atri
14. squam
15. son

16. aud
17. aur
18. script
19. barb
20. ped
21. bucc
22. cale
23. radi
24. quinque and par
25. pur
26. ros
27. calc
28. ur
29. cap
30. capill
31. seb
32. rig
33. cerebr
34. rub
35. cret
36. ocul
37. magn
38. line
39. later
40. lacrim
41. junct
42. jacul
43. hes
44. gingiv
45. gen
46. fus
47. furc
48. fun
49. foll
50. fiss
51. lact
52. fact
53. ego and path
54. lev and duct
55. dextr
56. dent
57. cut

58. cuss
59. cusp

Part E
1. semi
2. prim or un
3. sesqui
4. bi or second
5. tri or terti
6. quadru or quart
7. quinque or quint
8. sext
9. sep or sept
10. oct
11. non
12. ten
13. cent
14. mil

Part F
1. viscer
2. articul
3. aur
4. bucc
5. call
6. cut or pell
7. capill and pil
8. cerebr
9. cervic and coll
10. cipit
11. cord
12. dent
13. digit
14. gen
15. gingiv
16. inguin
17. labi
18. lien
19. mamm and pector
20. man
21. ment
22. nar

23. nas
24. nerv
25. nev
26. ocul
27. os and or
28. oss
29. ped
30. pulmon
31. ren
32. vent

Chapter 5
Part A
1. dysarthia
2. apophysis
3. eubiotics
4. dystrophy
5. aphasia
6. exocardiac
7. cataplexy
8. antipruritic
9. hypergia
10. ecmnesia
11. peripheral
12. paraplegia
13. endocrine
14. epidemic
15. excrement
16. esodic
17. parafibular
18. anastalsis
19. epidermis
20. asymmetrical
21. prognosis
22. antibiotic
23. anastomosis
24. hypogastropagus
25. euhydration
26. anesthetic
27. amphogenic
28. apoplexy
29. hypophrenia

Part A—cont'd

30. environment
31. pericranium
32. metabiosis
33. hyperergy
34. embryo
35. symbiosis
36. prosdonthia
37. progeria
38. exocrine

Part B

1. to change or to transfer
2. both
3. toward or addition to
4. within
5. beside or associated with
6. outward or outside
7. normal
8. into or inward
9. before
10. not or without
11. both
12. more
13. away
14. external
15. up or again
16. inward
17. down or against
18. less
19. within
20. not or without
21. with or together
22. upon
23. external
24. around or nearby
25. bad or difficult
26. outward or outside
27. inward
28. opposite
29. into or inward
30. inward

Part C

1. condition wherein both eyes are turned downward
2. cell layer lining the blood vessels and organs
3. less than normal number of digits
4. around the bronchus
5. inserted below the skin
6. webbed fingers
7. above the ear
8. inability to write properly
9. protein marker on cells which denote "self" or "not self"
10. paralysis resulting from stroke
11. within the heart
12. branch of psychiatry; study of what happens outside the brain
13. branch of dentistry; tooth extraction
14. marriage outside of ones own group
15. removal of water
16. the ability to remember
17. the ability to live without oxygen
18. pertaining to the brain
19. brain cell
20. mentally turning others away
21. outer layer of skin on an embryo
22. permanent kidney
23. relieving paralysis
24. satellite cell
25. ability to live on land and water
26. disease which is spread by personal contact
27. displacement of an internal part; hernia
28. inside the eye
29. hormone secretion from some place other than a gland
30. incorrect color perception
31. skin eruption
32. removal of the brain
33. normal condition of bile
34. normal concentration of glucose in the blood
35. any one event in a sequence
36. an agent which prevents disease
37. pertaining to the anterior part of the head
38. absence of a heart
39. absence of a head
40. rapid breathing
41. rapid frequent talking
42. excessive mental activity

Part D

1. translucid
2. infrared
3. succursal
4. prescription
5. subaqueous
6. obfuscation
7. ultrastructure
8. contraceptive
9. haematobic
10. subapical
11. intercrescence
12. projectile
13. dissect
14. ultrasound
15. introcession
16. retronasal

17. percussion
18. retrography
19. proliferate
20. interarticular
21. circumference
22. suppository
23. juxa-articular
24. post cardial
25. antecedent
26. resection
27. excrement
28. superscription
29. circumvent
30. preclusion
31. intravenous
32. postnasal
33. transverse
34. inappetence
35. perfussion
36. intraoccular
37. complicate
38. suffusion
39. external
40. secernment
41. respiration
42. califacient
43. secrete
44. ambidexterous
45. impalpable
46. prognosis
47. conjectiva
48. postmortem
49. insult

Part E
1. backward or back
2. from
3. across
4. under or somewhat
5. beyond
6. with
7. between or among

8. out or complete
9. on the side or close to
10. out or complete
11. near or toward
12. forward or in front of
13. below
14. out or complete
15. under or somewhat
16. above
17. before
18. around
19. with
20. near or toward
21. across
22. within
23. toward or complete
24. above
25. backward
26. opposite
27. apart
28. under or somewhat
29. into
30. into
31. apart
32. through or wrong
33. again
34. within
35. toward or complete
36. near or toward
37. both
38. before
39. backward
40. toward or complete
41. apart
42. with
43. after or behind
44. again
45. away
46. under or somewhat
47. near or toward
48. both
49. across

Part F
1. to bend backward
2. cessation of milk production
3. period just before the diastolic in the heart cycle
4. ability to move the thumb toward other digits
5. after tissue death
6. through the skin
7. during childbirth
8. across the eye
9. pertaining to breathing
10. to write within
11. to draw together
12. absorption of a liquid
13. below the heart area
14. unable to copulate
15. pertaining to sounds inaudible by the human ear
16. absence of arms
17. between the atria of the heart
18. to throw outward
19. across a wall (of tissue)
20. to throw across
21. prior to a fevers onset
22. in front of the head
23. to cut around
24. below the collar bone
25. opposite side
26. pertaining to the area above the ear
27. pertaining to the back of the head

Chapter 6
Part A
1. optician
2. physician
3. polycystic

Part A—cont'd

4. synthetic
5. psoriasis
6. heteradena
7. arthralgia
8. pathogenic
9. cryptogenic
10. bilirubinemia
11. hypophrenia
12. mastectomy
13. biarticulate
14. carbohydrate
15. ovary
16. mammary
17. malary
18. ampigean
19. metacarpal
20. chondrosteral
21. topical
22. genetics
23. presbyatrics
24. pediatrics
25. multigravida
26. primagravida
27. translucid
28. saline
29. hyaline
30. adiposis
31. secundines
32. meniscus
33. bronchitis
34. phlebismus
35. phlebotomist
36. halitosis
37. acromastitus
38. epithelium
39. endothelium
40. perinephrium
41. bacterium
42. chorditis
43. stomion
44. decimeter

45. gonometry
46. gonometer
47. cauterize
48. anastomosis
49. sarcoma
50. astronomy
51. condyloma
52. hyaloid
53. iridochoroiditis
54. psychiatrist
55. terminology
56. syndesmology
57. pyretolysis
58. phleboclysis
59. edema
60. exanthema
61. nacromania
62. centimeter
63. meglomania

Part B

1. fear of
2. surgical opening of
3. remedy for or by
4. to make or to treat
5. loving
6. in shape of
7. study of
8. study of
9. measure
10. means for placement
11. member or person
12. dissolution by
13. consequence/result of
14. formation of
15. process by which
16. loving
17. in shape of
18. process by which
19. madness/insanity about
20. placement for
21. one who/that which

22. consequence/result of
23. little
24. disease of
25. chemical derivative of
26. process by which
27. chemical derivative of
28. full of/pertaining to
29. little
30. one who/that which
31. condition affecting urine
32. surgery on or by
33. pertaining to or like
34. condition of
35. process by which
36. remedy for or by
37. pertaining to or like
38. one who
39. one who
40. related to
41. tumor resulting from/contained within
42. condition of
43. study of measure
44. inflammation of
45. related to
46. characterized as being diseased
47. part of or little
48. pertaining to or like
49. pertaining to or like
50. abnormal flow
51. little
52. to make
53. removal of
54. condition affecting blood
55. state of
56. state of
57. one who specializes in
58. pertaining to
59. pertaining to or like
60. related to

Part C

1. rotate
2. quarternate
3. error
4. cardiopulmonary
5. gastropulmonary
6. mammary
7. bigeminy
8. unicellular
9. tumor
10. parafibular
11. horny
12. malignant
13. ambulance
14. pregnancy
15. appearance
16. tonus
17. substance
18. motor
19. inappetency
20. vessel
21. clivius
22. incisor
23. intracutaneous
24. temperature
25. subcutaneous
26. septimal
27. callous
28. rupture
29. punctual
30. adrenal
31. dysbulia
32. efficacious
33. nervous
34. momentum
35. fibrous
36. magnitude
37. fulcrum
38. excrementitious
39. quadralivent
40. capacious
41. cerebellum
42. excrement
43. furuncle
44. sebaceous
45. impalpable
46. pilosebaceous
47. penduculus
48. tentaculum
49. aptitude
50. diotic
51. susceptible
52. mammalia
53. carbuncle
54. organelle
55. regimen
56. exophthalmic
57. areola
58. specimen
59. testicle
60. purulent
61. specula
62. stable
63. melantrichous
64. vitrification
65. ventricle
66. refractive
67. translucid
68. vitamin
69. pluriparity
70. connective
71. motile
72. ventrose
73. ossify
74. luminosity
75. tussive
76. nariform
77. incoherent
78. funiculus
79. involvcrum
80. absorption
81. varicose
82. labile
83. rigid
84. bistratose
85. tubercle
86. filiform
87. resection
88. lancet
89. tactile
90. erosion
91. projectile
92. suppository
93. optic
94. tremulous
95. mitochondria
96. systole
97. incidence
98. confluent
99. fibril
100. rigidity
101. venule
102. arciform
103. ambulatory
104. febrile
105. amnesia
106. nodule
107. erugatory
108. spectrum
109. incandescence
110. irrigate
111. afferent

Part D

1. able to
2. pertaining to
3. state or quality of being
4. pertaining to
5. to be
6. pertaining to
7. pertaining to
8. characterized as being
9. resulting from; act of; placement of
10. resulting from; act of; placement of

Part D—cont'd

11. small
12. means of; resulting from
13. resulting from; act of
14. pertaining to
15. to drive
16. small
17. small
18. small
19. small
20. state or quality of being
21. to be
22. full of
23. to begin or somewhat
24. small
25. state or quality of being
26. to make or to cause
27. having the shape of
28. to make or cause
29. state or quality of being
30. pertaining to
31. to be
32. able to
33. pertaining to
34. inclination toward
35. to be
36. to drive
37. small
38. pertaining to
39. small
40. small
41. pertaining to
42. resulting from; act of
43. full of
44. characterized as having
45. characterized by
46. state of; able to
47. state or quality of being
48. inclination toward
49. small
50. full of; predisposed to
51. resulting from; act of
52. resulting from; act of
53. resulting from; act of
54. small
55. small
56. one who; state of; resulting from
57. inclination toward; placement for
58. full of
59. full of
60. pertaining to
61. means of; resulting from
62. state or quality of being
63. pertaining to
64. small
65. inclination toward
66. small
67. small
68. small
69. small
70. inclination toward
71. resulting from; act of
72. resulting from; act of
73. state of being; act of doing

Chapter 7
Part A

1. Used to remove loose tissue from body surfaces. Clay, oatmeal, powder, rice, pumice, aluminum oxides, and salt are included in the category. Also called an exfoliate.
2. Products that break up or disband other substances.
3. Used as a food preservative. Vinegar is found in this category.
4. Crystal used in microdermabrasion.
5. A surfactant found in shampoos, cleansers, and body washes.
6. A surfactant that is more irritating than ammonium laureth sulphate.
7. Vitamins and substances that prevent free-radical formation; vitamins A, C, and E are found in this category.
8. An element that has a pleasant fragrance.
9. Vitamin C; contains antioxidant and skin-lightening components.
10. A topical product used to clarify the skin; restores the natural acidity of the skin.
11. A tree resin used for healing and soothing
12. An effective preservative, especially against molds and yeast.
13. A bactericidal agent used in acne care.
14. An effective preservative used against bacteria.
15. Derived from carrot oil; contains antioxidant and photo-protection properties.
16. Associated with herbs
17. Mild astringent with cooling qualities; used to relieve itching.
18. A naturally occurring chalk found in limestone; also found in coral and marble. Used in toothpastes and other personal products.

19. Used to create a red-orange color in cosmetic formulations.
20. Found in cosmetics, assist in reducing transepidermic water loss (TEWL).
21. An antioxidant and astringent from citrus fruits.
22. Properly called *cocamidopropyi dimethyl glycine*, this member of the betaine family is used as a mild-foaming and cleansing agent to reduce the irritancy of harsher surfactants in shampoos.
23. Found in skin, cartilage, and other connective tissues; gives the skin support and a youthful appearance.
24. Nontoxic element; has a catalytic action for keratinization and is considered a trace element in topical preparations. May also play a role in the formation of collagen by promoting certain enzymatic activities.
25. A herb used to purify the blood.
26. Contains antibacterial properties; seems to shorten the healing time of skin lesions.
27. Topical ingredient found in cosmetic preparations for the purpose of moisturizing.

28. Helps enhance smoothness and flexibility of the skin when used in a topical cosmetic preparation.
29. Reduces surface tension; used in cosmetic preparations to bind soluble oil and water ingredients.
30. Organic catalyst produced by cells to create chemical reactions; breaks up food and synthesizes proteins in the digestive process for body use.
31. Inorganic substance that is added to toothpaste to prevent decay.
32. A product that kills fungi.
33. Popular humectant used in moisturizers; binds water.
34. An agent used to retain moisture.
35. A component of glycosaminoglycans and a natural component of the skin.
36. A common process during which water and a salt produce a product with an acid and a base. Conversion of protein to amino acids in the digestive process is a common occurrence.
37. Derived from coconut oil; an emollient and moisturizer.

38. Used in skin care products as an emollient, moisturizer, and preservative; an alpha hydroxy acid
39. Phospholipid delivery device used in skin care products.
40. An important element in enzyme reactions; contributes to amino acid synthesis.
41. A silicone used in cosmetic powders.
42. Vitamin B3
43. Vitamin B
44. Para-amino benzoic acid; a water-soluble acid found in B vitamins; used as a sunscreen; can be an irritant.
45. Vitamin B5; a moisturizer.
46. Papaya enzyme found in pineapples; used as an exfoliate.
47. A lubricant and an emollient; an occlusive agent.
48. Used to adjust a product's pH.
49. An alpha hydroxy acid; derived from sodium pyruvate; has a very large molecule.
50. Used for conditioning the skin; more mild than retinoic acid.
51. Used as a peel solution; has a strong keratolytic activity; digests the debris in follicles; good for acne care.

Part A—cont'd

52. Synthetic detergent commonly used in shampoos and cleansers.

Part B

1. retinoid
2. one drop
3. melanin
4. to create chemical or enzyme reactions
5. prophylaxis
6. toxicology
7. a reaction involving oxygen
8. endorphins
9. anaerobic
10. sporicide
11. lipoprotein
12. contaminant
13. melanoma
14. keratin
15. three times a day
16. as occasion requires
17. adverse reaction
18. narcotic
19. hormone
20. electrolyte
21. contamination
22. a centrifuge
23. btu or calorie
24. Pandemic
25. endocrine glands

Index